The Way : Knowledge Balances Territory and Compassion

PHILLIP C. GIOIA, MD, MPH

THE WAY : KNOWLEDGE BALANCES TERRITORY AND COMPASSION

INFORMATION CONQUERS WASTE

2008

The Way : Knowledge Balances
Territory and Compassion

TABLE OF CONTENTS

THE DISCUSSION CONTINUES

For corrections, suggestions and addendums please e-mail me, Phillip Gioia. If you permit I will attach your contributions to future electronic copies of this hypertext.

Secure e-mail at www.RelayHealth.com—a free registration is required. Insecure e-mail drgioia@verizon.net

Web site with general health information and contacts— http://pages.prodigy.net/pcgioia

For the latest copy of the book please call or visit or mail my office 315-253-6257 at 37 W. Garden St., Auburn, NY 13021. $25 for book on floppy disc and $35 on paper manuscript or online from www.Amazon.com. Copyright 2006 by Phillip C Gioia

*This Book Is Dedicated To My Adaptive Parents
Rose And J. Charles Gioia.*

INTRODUCTION TO THE WAY

This is a book to help individuals and groups to feel better in a sustainable way. By using knowledge from the past and present we will help ourselves, help others and thereby help our species and its home, our planet. Since the origins of vertebrates territory has been used as a way to divide resources among individuals and families in a species. Humans have homes and yards often still. Since the origins of vertebrates compassion has been used to protect the immature and frail members of a species. Humans still tend to be attracted to and give to children and the ill. These feelings touch deep powerful emotions that may be used to motivate us to help our species or may be used to manipulate us to divert resources to harming our species. Since the origins of primates and before, species have developed social groups with their own leaders ruling over territories and providing for the immature and helpless. With symbols, language and ideas territory and compassion have often become abstract. We have resources in banks in our virtual territory of an account or in corporations in shares. We show our compassion by bank or stock transfers to charitable institutions. We even claim ideas as territory with copyrights and patents. Nations and international organizations identify with territories of demarcated lands or the whole planet. Groups may claim the ideal of territory or compassion as their own territory. Nations and/or regional organizations often combine their traditional geographic territory and their compassion for their residents or group members to be especially powerful at motivating their members. This may help our species adapt to our local, regional and global environment or this may just satisfy some of our primitive emotions to the short term benefit of some greedy territorial leader. With knowledge of our history, our psychology, our biology, our sociology and our economics in the past and in real time in the present we are better able to determine what is best for our species and ourselves. In the past we depended on bureaucrats and academics to guide us. Now information in corporation systems and on the Internet is more up to date and accurate than the 19th century built infrastructures of knowledge. Corporations may use this information to their advantage in lobbying and marketing. The public and its government must use it to benefit our society and species.

In a capitalistic materialistic society compassion is often sought as a spiritual oasis. Helping the immature, the sick and the needy does help us feel good about ourselves and help our species by promoting its survival with diverse individuals with their own special skills. Religions, political groups and nations that strive for this alone ultimately become victim to extremes of territory. Only groups that recognize the need for resources and know how to accumulate them will continue to exist. The protective cover of altruism or compassion then may allow the leaders and bureaucracy to accumulate immense wealth to the sole benefit of the hierarchy.

Similarly in a socialistic communistic society territory is often sought as a practical oasis. Rewarding creative and productive workers and developers helps us all improve our physical lives. Individuals, corporations, and multinational corporations that recognize only the material world may accumulate much wealth while harming the environment and social structures. If we recognize the territorial and compassionate needs and accept them in our organization and ourselves then we will better control them, and use these emotions to keep our organizations and ourselves self-sustaining and helpful to our species and ourselves.

Now in our political, energy, environmental and health crisis's we have one complex solution to help the species and its members. Knowledge of our past and present will guide us to the way to live. For most of us in most areas this means using non-violence to work with others with limited use of force for prudent self-defense as needed. We should use our own muscle power for energy and exercise when possible with renewable energy sources to supplement as needed and non-renewable sources only as an efficient investment in a self-sustaining future. Whole vegetables, fruits, nuts, and grains should be our main sources of food to help decrease our energy, land, and health needs. With less energy use, less disease and less pollution our political problems will be easier to solve. Using whole foods derived from plants for our main food source will decrease our main problems of heart disease and cancer. With less waste on wars and animal protein production we will be able to give more resources to the poor and needy of our nation and the world. This will make the world safer from extremism, infectious disease and violence while giving a better social and health environment to all. With "the devil in the detail" we must use our information systems to administer, monitor and control these massive yet essential changes to avoid the excesses of compassion creating dependence and waste; and the excesses of greed creating huge territories or fortunes with little benefit for the species. To survive humans must adapt and to do it well we need powerful transparent yet secure and private information systems.

SECTION I.
Need 2 Know/Hide

CHAPTER 1
Visions of Knowledge/Ignorance: Smallpox Scenarios

#1 The Present or Recent Past-

The United States of America (USA) is just starting to vaccinate military and medical frontline responders to smallpox. Many people with fever and hard white bumps on their arms and legs start appearing in the Midwest. Alert physicians and nurses suspect smallpox and immediately isolate the sick and contact the Centers for Disease Control and Prevention for a definitive diagnosis (http://www.bt.cdc.gov/agent/smallpox/overview/disease-facts.asp). The diagnosis is made within 24 hours. All known contacts are vaccinated within the next 2 days. Overseas reports of smallpox cases start to come in. Simultaneously a massive attack on the Internet by computer viruses shuts down the Internet for a few hours and slows down communication for days. Cases continue in contacts that were not vaccinated and containment of new cases is again done with immunization with smallpox vaccine of contacts of the new cases. In communities with many cases smallpox vaccine is offered to everyone. About 30% of the smallpox patients die. About 1% of the vaccinated contacts that have poor immune systems or severe eczema will die. Many are severely ill and some become disabled with brain and eye damage. Overseas the disease spreads in the poorly developed countries of the world where the health care resources are limited. The World Health Organization (WHO) begins to mount an effort to contain and eliminate smallpox once again as in the 1970's. Many people die and suffer but information about many individuals and organizations is on paper and thus inaccessible except at its storage site.

#2 The Future with Improved Knowledge and Security Systems -

The United States of America (USA) has finished its final phase of voluntary smallpox vaccination. A few people with fever and a hard white rash on their arms and legs start appearing in the Midwest. Alert physicians and nurses suspect smallpox and immediately isolate the sick and contact the Centers for Disease Control and Prevention [http://www.bt.cdc.gov] for a definitive diagnosis. The Health and Security Network (HaSN) quickly determines that all the people with the rash lack any smallpox vaccination within the past 10 years. The definitive diagnosis is made within 24 hours. The HaSN electronic records of death in a nearby area of the Midwest show a cluster of smallpox deaths at the same time. Using secure HaSN instant messages, phone messages, or home visits; local public health workers immediately contact all people that were close to the patients sick with smallpox that lack vaccination. The HaSN is used to rapidly find all the non-vaccinated contacts. At the same time their local health departments and health care providers are notified by the HaSN to plan for vaccination within the next day. Few people die since contact vaccination is complete within the crucial first two days after contact. There are few cases after the initial ones. This limits the number of vaccines that need to be given to people with poor immune systems or severe eczema.

With the use of the HaSN the untreated people that died with smallpox at home were found to be a group of people that often associated. People that sometimes dealt with them noted that had an extreme admiration for living things including viruses. A new computer virus is unleashed shutting down the non-secure Internet for days. The HaSN easily copes with the computer virus using traps and limited access to its registered computers. With the HaSN records, members of the group who traveled overseas were tracked and the information given to the WHO (World Health Organization) and the health agencies of the countries of travel. Immunization of contacts is begun immediately and members of this group promoting the smallpox virus are isolated to prevent further spread of the smallpox. The group members that volunteered to carry the smallpox used veils, scarves, hoods and winter masks to avoid people noting their typical smallpox rash. Access to the HaSN is limited on a strict need to know basis so that neighbors and friends will be unaware of group associations or medical treatments unless a criminal charge is brought against a person.

#3 The Future with a Comprehensive Knowledge and Security Integrated System -

The United States of America with the United Nations (UN) has just implemented its International Health and Security Network (IHaSN). Computer hackers from a small area of the Midwest have been attempting to break into the world smallpox reserve computer security system. The hackers plan to authorize smallpox virus for research work with a new anti-viral medicine to be done at the Centers for Disease Control and Prevention (CDC) in the USA. The CDC's last batch was destroyed to help decrease security problems and costs. Associates of the hackers have been contacting foreign governments and groups hostile to the USA to try to buy smallpox virus to use to spread the disease. They say they want to destroy the USA. The FBI/CIA cooperative and Interpol do investigation. The fingerprints used for the Internet access and the computer identification codes match those of friends and community members associated with people in the underground Virus Liberation Movement (VLM). Secure Internet access at this time requires a fingerprint reader, user identification, and a matching secure personal identification number (PIN) using a registered computer.

At the same time the group has used the identities of their unsuspecting others to make phone and letter contacts. All phone calls at this time require an electronic user identification number and a matching PIN. Letters require a unique barcode for the sender along with an encoded PIN. Receiver addresses are also bar-coded. Postal computers record and track all mail and parcels. Receivers may block letters from some addresses, and for security may only accept mail or parcels from senders who also know their special receiver PIN and have it encoded on the letter or parcel.

The VLM plans to release smallpox back into the environment. This will help let the virus reach its full potential. They also plan to release large number of computer viruses into the electronic environment. These will be blocked from all registered computers on the state protected International Health and Security Network by anti-virus traps and programs within the network. The Virus Liberation Movement hopes to attack the wild old Internet remnants and the unvaccinated of the world to let the viruses live. The VLM gained access to registered and secure computers of unsuspecting friends and acquaintances.

By the time the VLM has found one rogue organization to give them the smallpox virus, Interpol has tracked them down and arrested them with the virus shipment. The smallpox release is prevented. Some at large members of the VLM upset at their failure with real viruses release the computer viruses into unregulated parts of the Internet causing damage to computer networks in developing countries without the latest computer virus protection. New secure identity cards are given to the unsuspecting associates of the VLM with stolen security access and identities, to prevent further breaches in their Internet, phone and postal security. VLM members who were against violence and helped to stop it are also given new identity cards to protect them from attacks by violent VLM members. Developed countries work to improve security in the developing world to help maintain international communication, health and commerce. Information on individuals and organizations is only shared as permitted by the responsible party and only to designated trusted receivers of the information. All countries, social groups, and individuals have the right to review or audit the detailed access history of their own records.

CHAPTER 2.
The Best Balance of Territory and Compassion

Which scenario would you like? Throughout the centuries of our existence there have been benefits to knowledge and to secrecy. There have also been many abuses of both. In this book I would like to review the history of knowledge and secrecy as used to help people, yet protect their territory. We will discuss past and present choices and make recommendations for future choices that may help our species and environment survive in the best possible state. Our species now must make major decisions regarding information processing. Our information technology revolution is forcing us to choose between an efficient and powerful connected information network with tremendous potential for benefits and abuses, or to continue with fragmented, disintegrated, redundant systems which will be hard to use and abuse. Both choices have benefits and dangers. How the choices are implemented will be very important. The integrated system must be strictly controlled and protected to prevent abuse by the powerful controllers of the system or from any possible intruders. With the integrated data system automated and high security review of data by a select few with explicit directives and limits determined by a legislative directive subject to judicial review would be best. With the continuation of our separate data systems trusted observers and regulators must constantly review the fragmented systems to make them useful at all for health and security. Our inability to use these separate data systems to prevent the 9/11 2001 terrorist attack, distribute influenza vaccine, and communicate when hit by natural disasters such as Hurricane Katrina, bode poorly for continuing this system in its present state. First I will briefly discuss the smallpox scenarios.

In the first scenario taking place in the present/ recent past, people with smallpox that present to physicians, will be detected at about the time the smallpox virus becomes infective. At the end of 2002 experts believe that the virus will unlikely spread to other casual contacts until the typical smallpox rash becomes easily visible during a routine examination by a physician or other well-trained health care provider. In the NBC TV show <u>ER</u> broadcast at the end of the spring 2002 season the smallpox virus was shown to spread to ER staff when the smallpox infected patient first got a fever 2 to 4 days before the typical rash appears. This sometimes occurs if the infected person shares food or drink or kisses another person (http://www.bt.cdc.gov/agent/smallpox/overview/disease-facts. asp). Most experts believe that smallpox infected patients with fever but without the rash would rarely transmit the smallpox virus to ER staff, healthcare workers, casual acquaintances or passersby. This is consistent with the ability to contain natural smallpox in the 1970's with programs that just vaccinated known contacts of the smallpox infected. Vaccinating contacts within 3 to 4 days of contact with the virus is able to prevent severe smallpox. The sooner the vaccination is done after contact the better. Vaccinating within 72 hours (3 days) of contact is most effective, but even up to 96 hours (4 days) still prevents most of the severe disease

(http://www.bt.cdc.gov/agent/smallpox/basics/index.asp). Even with this limited period of contagion tracking the path of an infectious person and finding all the contacts is very daunting in our mobile society, especially if the person was contagious while in a school, concert, church, subway, train station, bus terminal or airport. If the person knowingly concealed the illness and tried to expose the maximum number of mobile people before dropping from the illness the task to vaccinate all exposed within 3 to 4 days of exposure would be nearly impossible. Our data systems on travel and contacts are insufficient to quickly document and find these contacts. We could only hope that the number of concealed ill was small and we soon discovered all the non-concealed cases and their contacts. At present we must plan on about 30% of the unvaccinated smallpox infected dying. This is the rational for the 2002 plan of President Bush to offer smallpox vaccination to the general public in the year 2004. This would cause 1/3 of the vaccinated to get ill enough to miss work in 7-10 days from the smallpox vaccine, 1 in 1000 people to become severely ill with hospitalization, and 1 in a million to die, but would protect the survivors for 10 years from a concealed exposure to smallpox.

Unless we know the future chance of smallpox exposure we are unable to accurately tell whether the risk of the vaccine is more or less than the risk of disease or death from smallpox. Only by gathering more information on smallpox, terrorists external/internal, travel, communications and resource or money flows will we better able to plan and prepare. To better survive and use our resources we must decrease the number of unknown variables. For a discussion of a proposed National Health Information Infrastructure [NHII] see the work of the National Committee on Vital and Health Statistics [NCVHS] web page (http://ncvhs.hhs.gov) and its report on the NHII (http://ncvhs.hhs.gov/nhiilayo.pdf). At the same time we must decrease the number variables known to the terrorists to make their actions and planning less successful. When we gather information it should just be available on a need to know basis with the high-level information systems protected by identification that is linked to unique body markers. These systems will take time and money but they will guard the health of the community and the privacy of the individuals. As at present for sensitive information on sexually transmitted diseases, inherited genetic tendencies, and behavior problems; security to prevent disclosure must be strong. Penalties for wrongful disclosure must be severe and enforced. When we spend time entering our identification codes, using our smart cards, swiping through bar codes, and then entering our PIN (personal identification code) and/or placing our fingerprints on a machine reader we must feel the information is used only for the good of the community and ourselves. When we need to enter a high security area or have a large money or property transfer we may need further levels of verification with perhaps pattern analysis of our face or iris (the biologic shutter around the pupils of our eyes). For the highest levels of security, pattern analysis of our retina (the back of our eye seen through our pupil) or DNA analysis may be necessary. Machines that communicate through the Internet, phone networks, and radio networks should be uniquely registered with identifiers hardwired into their silicone chips. Intel tried to do this with computers a few years before September 11, 2001 causing a huge outcry from those afraid of losing their privacy. When knowledge for public protectors becomes critical to our survival we should reconsider this option. Computers, phones, cell phones, radios, PDA's (personal data assistants) and all communicating machines or appliances with phone, radio or Internet connections should be identified. Again public information stores must guarded with information just available with a need to know basis. Parents of young children might have access to know their whereabouts and activities, but neighbors or friends would have none unless explicitly granted by the person or their guardian. I am sure that on reading this, most of our USA citizens would think this would never happen due to the extreme right to privacy in the USA. Many might think it would be helpful to the public good but would never get enough political support to come about. Of course some would rather get smallpox and die than give their acquaintances any chance of learning about parts of their lives that they want hidden. This is often related to a deep need of many to be protected from shame. I believe that with proper protections against terrorists, unauthorized access, strict redundant security, and absolute privacy for individual matters and feelings that have little effect on the community; a comprehensive information system may work and be politically acceptable in the USA. Even the staunch supporter of civil rights and privacy, Harvard Law Professor, author and crusader Alan Dershowitz would support a national identifier system if it were done correctly (http://www.law.harvard.edu/faculty/directory/facdir.php?id=12). He discusses this in his book Why Terrorism Works (2002). He would rather have people being investigated intelligently based on accurate and meaningful information rather than broad categories now used for police surveillance profiling such as race, dress, ethnicity or type of car driven. In that same book Professor Dershowitz discusses when it might be necessary and socially acceptable to resort to torture to prevent mass catastrophes. Better data systems would help prevent the possible use of torture that causes shame in our souls of compassion and civility and often produces questionable results.

At present we are ill prepared for another internal attack as the Oklahoma City Bombing by Tim McVeigh in April

1995 (http://www.cnn.com/US/OKC/bombing.html). Our only improvement in surveillance is the temporary legislation known as the USA Patriot Act of 2002 and its 2006 extension allowing the FBI to examine credit card records. This may easily be circumvented by using credit cards that are stolen or with false identities. The recent credit card theft ring in Long Island demonstrates how easy and lucrative this practice is (http://www.utica.edu/academic/institutes/cimip/about/uc.cfm). Clearly for homeland and financial security we need better identification financial and legal transactions. Similarly we must be able to identify the smallpox virus's spreaders. Often false identities are used for health insurance fraud (http://www.cms.hhs.gov/FraudAbuseforConsumers/) or to avoid embarrassment by involvement in the diagnosis and treatment of sexually transmitted disease or psychiatric illness or private family matters (http://www.connectingforhealth.org/commonframework/). To protect confidentiality we might allow patients to have multiple identities so that they would be comfortable getting essential lifesaving medical care without the fear of losing their privacy. For national security purposes each identity would be connected in the highest security area of the national integrated database. Friends, neighbors, community members, employers and insurers would lack any access to the linked data. If a person had a diagnosis of smallpox, anthrax, Human Immunodeficiency Virus (HIV) or other contagious deadly disease only public health and law enforcement investigators at the highest security levels would be able to link the data. We are better prepared for foreign attacks by screenings at airports, border crossings and customs, though passports can too easily be stolen or forged. Automobile driver's licenses have similar limitations. Both might be improved with the use of a smart card with coded information on personal information with access only through a PIN and fingerprint, facial pattern or iris pattern recognition. For high security purposes the information could be verified on line from a secure data repository within seconds. This online check would verify that the person wanting to use a high security transportation, building or gain access to secure information was presently authorized to do so and free of any public health, financial, or criminal risk to others. For privacy the security personnel would only be given information on the need to know basis. So a person with HIV would certainly be free to travel on public transportation but if giving blood the blood bank computer would be told privately that the blood would be discarded without any one at the donor location or blood bank having to know the reason. Friends and acquaintances at the blood site would lack any access to the information. If the person being screened is found to have a warrant for a violent crime then local security personnel may be quietly informed of pertinent details and best plan for decreasing the risk to all the public at the location. The present USA passports are much more secure than in the past but other countries use passports that are still easy to modify or forge.

The developing countries of the world without our health care and information infrastructure will be hard hit if smallpox escapes to their populations. The resources of WHO (The World Health Organization) and the developing countries will be severely challenged. Smallpox might smolder for years in these countries with large disruptions occurring in health, culture, travel, transportation, and commerce that are all now global in many ways. To cope with these challenges developing countries with foreign aid as needed might develop simple efficient integrated data systems based on affordable technology that would best direct limited resources and help development. As hardware and wireless technology costs fall developing countries without wires may use open source software such as Linux or Google's to fill the information void with public systems that are easily usable, secure, and affordable. International agreements would be needed to share information on a need to know basis. Data would be kept within each country and only given to computers in other countries when the person travels. Contagious disease or criminal history may then preclude certain activities or travel but only officials who must be involved in risk reduction would be informed of the nature of the problem. Trusted ethical world leaders would be rewarded with information to help them deal with fanatic violent local individuals and groups.

In the second scenario we have implemented better tracking of people traveling on public transportation and using health services. Public health organizations are then better able to find contacts of infectious disease and prevent further spread of the disease. Police organizations are then better able to find the criminals spreading the disease and limit their criminal impact. The second scenario however lacks the means to effectively prevent disease and crime.

In the second scenario criminals, terrorists, pranksters, and hooligans are still allowed to use electronic and mail communications to perpetrate their damage to our society. We would likely continue to have bomb threats causing disruptions to businesses and schools. In NY State laws have been passed with severe penalties for such behavior with little help. The present mail system, that continues to use much of the same formal security that Ben Franklin gave it in the 1700's without the informal security provided by the all knowing local postmasters, lends itself to spreading disease and dangerous materials. Computer viruses, fraud, pornography, Internet attacks and electronic junk mail or spam clog the Internet making it more difficult and expensive to use for legitimate individuals and businesses. Our electronic world now is like the Wild West of the USA in the mid 1800's where people must defend themselves. The Bush Administration in October 2002 says that private corporations and individuals must provide for their own security (http://www.landfield.com/isn/ mail-archive/2002/Sep/0083.html , http://www.whitehouse. gov/pcipb).

This is a necessity at present, but lacks efficiency and effectiveness. Even the most conservative and liberal agree that government has an essential role in police protection. Since our future is in electronic information and commerce, government must police and regulate this environment. We accept the rules of the road and vehicle regulations for our bicycles, motorcycles, cars and trucks. Why fight them for our Internet communications and commerce? We accept being taxed to pay for our streets, roads, and superhighways. Why fight them for our information byways and superhighways that will make our country and world safer and more efficient? We accept the need to register motorcycles, cars, trucks, and buses. Why fight the registration of connected electronic devices such as phones, PDA's (personal digital assistants), and computers that might bring schools, businesses, or the defense department to disaster? We license and regulate professionals and businesses that are located in our state. Why fail to provide secure identification and licensing for them when they operate electronically in our home, commercial, and public networks? We prevent pollution of world with contagious disease and toxic substances. Why allow our machines for knowledge and business to be infected and damaged thereby threatening our health and economics? Just as we have set up infrastructures in the earth environment for communication, travel, transportation, economics and health we must also set up infrastructures in the electronic environment. Few of us would accept phones, train, airlines, or mail systems that fail to interact. Why do we accept failures in accounting systems, medical record systems, immigration and criminal justice systems that then fail to protect us from fraud, contagious disease, larceny, injuries and violent crime because of their inability to communicate securely to the public servants that need to know?

Bill Gates in <u>Business @ the Speed of Thought</u> on business information systems (<u>http://www.microsoft.com/billgates/speedofthought</u>) and Alvin Toffler in <u>POWERSHIFT</u> <u>http://www.amazon.com/exec/obidos/ASIN/0553292153/ref=ase_thewhythingsdont/104-0213690-2499931#product-details</u> believe that easy access to knowledge at anytime and anyplace is a key to our future well being. Bill Gates simply sees knowledge as essential to good management and business practices. Alvin Toffler sees knowledge as the key at present to controlling society. Knowledge as communicated will influence social choices and also makes the other means of social control: violence and wealth, more effective. Both see that we must progress beyond the period of mass production, mass religion, and bureaucracy to more flexible organizations through which information flows freely to where it is needed. Bill Gates sees within organization e-mail as helping out. He accepts e-mails from anyone in Microsoft and uses the information to make his organization better. From the anti-trust trouble he got into by writing down in his e-mail his ideas on eliminating Microsoft's competition, he probably needs to appreciate more the need to conceal. The e-mail archives were used against him and Microsoft in the government's anti-trust case involving the Windows operating system. Windows also lacks protections to attacks by viruses and worms. These illustrate the need for Microsoft to hide information from raiders of their territory. Alvin Toffler notes that informal social contacts and structures as among Japanese executives that start training in their corporation in the same year also help spread knowledge in corporations. The failure of the USA intelligence agencies to prevent the 9/11 2001 attack may in part be blamed on the lack of such broad electronic or informal means of communication. MIT (Massachusetts Institute of Technology) researchers found that information workers with active e-mail contacts were more productive   http://ebusiness.mit.edu/research/briefs.html.   Of course without appropriate security electronic communications might be used against the USA by terrorists gaining special information that show weaknesses in our defenses or by spreading misinformation. For our health and security we need more offensive (promoting physical and financial health), and defensive (protecting people and groups) information and must block terrorists and criminals from access to useful information.

To change our private and public sectors to be more adaptive with the use of new information and knowledge systems will take much time, money and political will. Bill Gates notes that even his huge corporation must avoid over reaching. Data and information systems should start with limited achievable goals. Bill Gates discusses at length the conflicts between the financial and information technology (IT) people within private organizations. Financial experts would like to see the IT departments make money or at least minimize their expenses. The IT people are usually a support service that contributes parts of functions to moneymaking parts of the organizations. Often it is difficult to account for how much income they produce for the corporation. Other departments that use them often wish to underestimate the value of IT to avoid sharing income with the IT department. MIT researcher Erik Brynjolfsson found that businesses investing in IT generally became more productive and those businesses adopting a digital organization became very productive within one to three years http://ebusiness. mit.edu/research/briefs.html. His group also found many IT failures for lack of education and planning. As a society we are poor at dealing with the value of ideas or intellectual property. Our Gross National Product (GNP) and our International Trade Deficit often fail to adequately account for income that we make on movies, music, and entertainment. Alvin Toffler notes that bureaucrats in businesses of the mass production orientation and in traditional government departments often control through limiting access to information in their departments to others. Information and analysis from these private or public departments is usually provided after a time delay, sometimes with special payments to the department, and often with view or opinions of the chief bureaucrat being built into the report. Accessible data and analysis systems available to other employees, stockholders or concerned citizens threaten the control of these bureaucrats.

Much of our evolution from vertebrates on to mammals and primates has involved territoriality. This allows for the allocation of resources for survival such as food and shelter. The territories serve to distribute species member individually or as in mammals in groups to certain areas that may support their growth and reproduction. Some of the bureaucratic and political behavior may be explained by this tradition. Often shame and pride mediate the protection of territories both physical and intellectual. Donald Nathanson in <u>Shame and Pride</u> explores in depth how we frequently use these affects and associated emotions subconsciously but fail to recognize them consciously(http://www.behavior.net/column/nathanson/bio.html). We know from infancy to have shame if we are unable to do some task. Often parents and/or teachers use this to control us as we grow. When shame becomes associated with guilt or emphasized in our early childhood we suffer pain whenever we experience shame. This often keeps us out of areas that bureaucrats would like to control. Those who are shame sensitive tend to stay within their own territory where they will make few errors, feel competent, are comfortable and have pride—our home. Unfortunately our world is changing rapidly and we now must often venture into new intellectual territory and real territory with travel. To deal with large problems such as natural disasters, terrorist attacks and large public events FEMA (Federal Emergency Management Agency) in DHS (Department of Homeland Security) has given us ways of creating administrative territory to deal with the situation called the Incident Command System (ICS) http://emilms.fema. gov/ . Only those who may tolerate failure and are willing to explore the unknown may go gladly into the future and adapt willingly. Much of our fear of computers and data systems is due to the shame we get when the machine or system fails to work as we expect it to. When systems become useful, stable, and easy to use and education in their use improves then even the faint of heart will take advantage of the new knowledge.

In the third scenario we have implemented the security in communication gaining the ability to prevent an attack on the public. Our danger now is in allowing the control over communications to protect those in power from the scrutiny of the public. Free speech must continue to be protected to give the public the ability to react to and correct the misuses of power. If electronic communications are properly used free speech may be increased. Computers may know who posts information; but only if there is a clear and present danger or definite intent to cause immediate harm, would the information be given to those with the highest security clearance. Cases that are uncertain or unclear or only might pose a future threat would be investigated after obtaining a confidential court order. On going surveillance would only be done with a warrant. Records of who has seen such private documents would be unalterable and maintained along with the documents. To facilitate this, copies of such records might be kept in the highest security areas in the administrative and judicial branches of government. With secure and accurate tamper proof records rogue elements both within and outside the government may be monitored and regulated by high security administrators and judiciary with legislative direction.

Another danger with knowing so much is in being forced to implement laws that many people are unable to obey. Our economy now depends on about 5 to 10 million illegal immigrants or aliens who do work that USA citizens avoid. Many farm laborers, restaurant workers, domestic workers, or heavy laborers come from other countries and work without current legal authority. We must incorporate them into our society legitimately by giving them some acceptable status. Illegal drugs and illegal drug dealers should be easier to track. We should provide treatments to drug users to help them avoid drug use. If we are still unable to cut the demand for these drugs to zero we may consider severely regulating and limiting the current illegal drugs to a limited legal distribution. We might then tax them and more easily prevent the drug profits from getting into the hands of terrorists and other criminals. Money from taxes might be used for drug use prevention and treatment of the addicted. This may also be applied to the abuse and addiction to legal drugs such as alcohol and tobacco. Treatments for users should be encouraged to reduce unhealthy use. Similarly the abuse of sexual contacts in prostitution, at home, in institutions or in spreading sexually transmitted diseases must be prevented and treated for the public protection. The sexually addicted should be treated to eliminate their destructive behavior and kept from vulnerable people if they may persist in the behavior. Public information systems may also be used for helping to prevent and treat nutrition and exercise problems. Confidential secure e-mail or phone calls may be used to help remind adults or parents of children with vitamin deficiencies, calorie or fat or protein excesses, or exercises deficiencies of the need to adjust their habits for better health.

Development of a secure health information system may help in solving the financial and quality crisis in health care and business. It also may provide for the key to providing quality health care for the uninsured. With a national health information system containing basic information on health care costs and health problems state governments may better analyze health problems and find health care that lacks/has cost effectiveness. Basically if we pay more for health care than its benefits are worth, we will have a net loss on health care. If we pay for health care that saves us money by decreasing future expenses for complications or preventable diseases, we will all gain. Government may then mandate cost effective care for all residents of our country with coverage through employment and/or taxes. With secure national health information systems, the responsible person will know before getting care what services or drugs will be covered. People or employers may opt for insurance or other coverage for health care services that lack proven cost effectiveness. A national board will continually review the art and science of medicine to provide coverage for new health care services that are shown to be cost effective and/or eliminate coverage for old services that are now shown to lack cost effectiveness in a new environment. At one time routine chest x-rays were cost effective when we had many people with tuberculosis in our country but as the number of people with the disease decreased the benefit of doing chest x-rays also decreased. In the future whole plant based food diets may be used to decrease heart disease, diabetes, cancer and diabetes. As evidence accumulates health care payers may promote programs that work in improving our diets. At present it is hard for businesses or insurance companies to manage such a program since many businesses change insurance companies year to year and many prevention programs only have a benefit over 5 to 10 years. For instance paying to help a 30 year olds to stop smoking costs money now but will give most benefits for decreasing heart disease risk over 1 year or more, and lung cancer risk over 5 years or more from the start of the program. A good health data system should also help decrease claim and administrative costs by helping to automate information processing and data exchange. Current insurance companies would be able to use the one state regulated system making it easier for health care providers to contact and communicate with the many insurance companies throughout the country. Just as in the other information sectors privacy must be protected. Health care providers and payers would be limited to get patient information on a strict need to know basis. Patients or there responsible caretaker would have to authorize patient information access to the health care provider. Providers would be protected from liability if only given incomplete information. Patients would have a secure identity (perhaps with a smart card) with a PIN and/or fingerprint confirmation for record access to be regulated by them and/or their caretaker.

Once basic public data systems in health, education, finance, government and security are working then information and knowledge may be used to improve better balance our territorial and compassionate needs. In healthcare, computers may be used to reduce errors in medications and diagnoses without threatening patients or healthcare providers. The Institute of Medicine (IOM) and the Agency for Health Care Research and Quality (AHRQ) have written extensively on how this might be done (http://www.ahcpr.gov/qual/errorsix. htm). Education achievement may be evaluated continually and resources directed as needed to help improve technical and social knowledge for the public, students, healthcare providers, administrators and politicians. Financial markets will be trustworthier with open and transparent accounting systems viewable by all yet secure and protecting privacy and identity. Government may measure citizen needs and resources in real time with improved responsiveness to the needs of individuals and communities without threatening beneficial adaptive local relations. Security systems will protect strategic information, crucial intellectual resources, critical geographic locations, and/or economics resources while allowing useful access to information to select individual or trusted organizations at the discretion of the individual or custodian. These systems may be combined in synergy to promote and monitor non-violence, energy conservation, exercise promotion, whole food plant derived diets, and a real defense of the resources of species and its home, our planet.

THE WAY TO BETTER WORLD HEALTH
SECTION II

Knowledge to Balance Compassion and
Territory in Health

CHAPTER 3
Know/Hide in Many Ways

There lots of ways to know/hide things. Often the knowledge we gain in different ways will lead to different conclusions. Judgment must be used to decide which knowledge to use and which to discount because of hidden or partial information. Given that the judgment process may be highly abstract and without concrete evidence of proof different people may come to different conclusions. This is the ultimate beauty of the USA with a Constitution enshrining freedom of information and choice. The founding fathers spent much on books and started the postal system even before the armed Revolution. This system allows me to write this book to help give the public an informed choice for their future. I believe that many people or even our whole species will be hurt or destroyed by poor information systems. I also believe that good information systems may be used to hurt or destroy many people or even our whole species if misused. As a public health physician I feel a duty to make sure that the public gets a chance to choose to develop safe and secure data systems that will best serve them. Now with data systems that are deficient to protect the public and allow the public to live in the best health possible with our limited economic resources I must inform my public health employer (administrators, politicians and ultimately the public) that my fellow public officials, citizens, residents and I may do better with a better information infrastructure. The evidence I present and my years of living in my family and community, and working in private and public health convinces me that to adapt to our world successfully we need a powerful yet secure and private information system. In reviewing the different forms of knowledge, I will describe the experience and information that I have used to come to this conclusion and why I judge it to be important.

I will review the knowledge/secrecy encoded in the biosphere, human genetics, religion, culture, specialists, data systems, feelings and direct individual experience. I will illustrate how we have used and misused knowledge in our quest for survival and health. I will discuss 10 major current public health problems that threaten our quality and quantity of life. With this information hopefully you will be able to distill the appropriate wisdom to deal with the foreseeable and unforeseeable futures.

These knowledge sources interact with our world and with each other. We may use these knowledge sources to help our species survive. Given a changing world an inflexible adaptation that works today may be a detriment to us tomorrow. Adaptations to one part of our world may help in that environment but may hinder in another part of our world. Immigration and migration make things even more complicated with environments changing rapidly as we move about the world and the old environment perhaps changing before we may get back to it. In our cultural life, in religion and in the graphic and performing arts we must also contend with virtual worlds as well as our physical world. Books, photography, film, automated sound production, sound recordings, digital presentations and the Internet have made the virtual world more malleable and instable compounding our speed of adaptation problem but giving the potential for adaptation that is responsive to the needs of individuals and the full potential of the species.

True knowledge and wisdom is more valuable to us than basic data or information that is often just given by our senses, our media, and our arts. Knowledge and wisdom will help guide us in the course of our life. Data or information just gives us representation of a small part of the world. Knowledge is what an experienced baseball manager such as Joe Torre uses to direct his team. Data on balls, strikes, hits and fielding help us find out what is happening. This raw data is processed into information such as batting averages and fielding percentages. The manager uses his experience with the information studied over different times and environments along with things outside the statistics like emotional and physical health to make the best decision possible about which players to use at which time. The good physician takes the data of temperature readings, blood pressures and weights then changes it into information by plotting the patterns over time. Using all the information on the patient including family and personal history the physician then decides if the patient has any significant problems and if any intervention is worth the trouble.

The biosphere takes the resources of energy and material substance to produce life. We humans are but a part of the biosphere or food web or circle of life. The biosphere adapts to changes in climate and chemicals with different mixes of species and interactions. Over long periods of time the species of the biosphere may adapt genetically to thrive in their niche of the environment. Jared Diamond in <u>Guns, Germs and Steel</u> has pointed out how Western Civilization was favored by a rich biosphere that was easy for humans to exploit by using easily domesticated plants to produce surpluses of grain such as wheat and rice and adapting large animals such as pigs, cows, chickens and horses to use for surpluses of protein for our diet and energy for building and transport. The grain and animals also adapted for a synergy of production with grains used for the animals and animal waste used to help the grain grow. We also benefited from cats protecting grain stores from rodents and dogs helping to manage grazing animals and protect us from large predators. The horses also helped in warfare for conquering other lands and protecting our homeland. Professor Diamond also shows that temperate Fertile Crescent of the Middle East was unique in its capability to produce such a fortuitous circumstance for Western Civilization. In this area of the world the viral disease small pox developed. Humans there adapted to it but when it naturally spread with Western Civilization other human groups often succumbed in large numbers. With time the presence of metal ores and fire brought on the production of steel that made further domination of the world possible through weapons such as swords and guns, and technology such as trains and modern ships   http://news.nationalgeographic.com/news/2005/07/0706_050706_diamond.html . This concatenation of energy and physical resources that produced a benevolent biosphere malleable by our capabilities is surely a great gift to Western Civilization. Of course just being on a planet that is able to sustain life is an amazing and rare circumstance. Hidden geography from the inner core of earth, to the ocean floor, to near planets, stars, and galaxies awaits future explorers. We must choose to protect our biosphere so that we are more likely to survive along with our biosphere co-inhabitants.

Human genetic knowledge/secrecy is built into our bodies. We are born with physical and mental attributes that help us gain resources from the world to grow and reproduce. Over thousands of years the genes of the species may be changed by the gradual selection of the ones that help us reproduce in the environment that has been present over many generations. This is the concept of genetic selection, evolution or Darwinism. This is a slow process since it takes many generations of breeding before the frequency of genes that help breeding are increased and those that inhibit breeding are decreased. This process of changing the genes in our species or gene pool is unable to adjust quickly to a rapidly changing world. Other sources of knowledge must be used to help us adjust our ways of living in order to survive with our given genetic qualities in our given environment. Though with genetic engineering, we may change this time frame drastically. If we chose to genetically engineer we must be sure that it will be for the best for it may have unforeseen implications for centuries.

Still hidden to us are the many parts and functions of genes. The human genome project tells use the chemical structure of our chromosomes but many long sections of the chromosomes have codes with unknown functions. We know chemicals called histones wrap around the chromosomes but we are unsure of their function in allowing the chromosomes to express themselves. We know the microenvironment of cells effects how the chromosomes function but only a few details are known. We know that mitochondria have their own genes with maternal inheritance but their role in health and disease is still being defined. With 30,000 different genes there are hundreds of millions of potentially significant gene interactions with most yet to be explored. The strong genetic drives to procreate are often hidden by religious and social values to avoid danger from disease and injury. These subconscious drives if uncontrolled may result in destruction and death with violence directed at others and the self.

In the United States of America at present we estimate that about 10% of the time disease is due to mainly genetics, about 10% of the time it is due to mainly environment, and to a mix of genetic and environmental factors about 80% of the time. For instance Down syndrome or Trisomy 21 is a strong genetic determinant of mental retardation and premature aging. Severe Lead Poisoning is a strong environmental determinant of mental retardation, seizures and anemia. Phenyl Ketonuria or PKU is a genetic problem in metabolizing the amino acid phenylalanine that will cause seizures and mental retardation when babies are fed normally but with a special diet low in phenylalanine the mental retardation and seizures are avoided. This was made possible by the work of many scientists including Dr. Robert Guthrie http://en.wikipedia.org/wiki/Robert_Guthrie.

In the developing world with poor water and food quality, environmental causes account for more of the disease burden. Using the following significant health information problems I will discuss how genetic and environmental factors interact to cause disease or promote health.

As genetics builds on the environment including the biosphere, so religion builds on our environment and our genetics. Religion helps us adapt to our surroundings and our inborn tendencies to help us survive. Religion is based on deeper truths and wisdom so it must be resistant to short term changes or distractions. Our tendency to believe stories and what authorities tell us, facilities believing in God and religion as Richard Dawkins expounds http://en.wikipedia.org/wiki/The_God_Delusion. At its best religion directs civilization toward success with productivity and enjoyment, though if ancient traditions fail to adapt to a changing world it may lead to behavior that is maladaptive to the present. Huge birth rates were definitely needed after the plague wiped out 1/3 of the population of Europe during the Middle Ages and probably made another 1/3 significantly depressed. Perhaps now religion might change toward more emphasis on quality of life with large populations of humans threatening our environment. Religions do change but very slowly. Christianity at its birth 2000 years ago, synthesized Jewish humanism, Zoroastrian common meals and the search for the truth and the light, Egyptian concepts of resurrection, Greek and Roman Goddess worship, and West African spirit walks http://en.wikipedia.org/wiki/Zoroastrianism. Joseph Campbell has written and talked about this much http://www.jcf.org/index2.php. Buddhism borrowed from Hinduism and the Muslims have built upon Jewish and Christian traditions. Given the human need to believe in something greater than our day-to-day existence and human fallibility, new religions or sects are constantly developing but only a few become successful. Karen Armstrong notes the importance of compassion in the religions of the Axial Age 2500 years ago http://en.wikipedia.org/wiki/Axial_Age. Compassion or empathy present in vertebrates and mammals to help with caring for the young (http://www.npr.org/templates/story/story.php?storyId=5534300) is newly emphasized in the Axial Age religions and philosophies of humanism http://www.npr.org/templates/story/story.php?storyId=5307044 . The development of iron weapons at that time stimulated a great deal of appreciation for non-violent techniques to conserve lives and resources. To survive more thought had to be given to conscious and subconscious ways to avoid unwise action and value human life. The core values of compassion and understanding in Christianity, Islam, Hinduism, Buddhism, and Taoism are often overcome by primitive vertebrate territorial impulses that bring violence back into religion. Religions when institutionalized become attached to local territories or nations and then justify violence to gain more resources for their special territory. Sects within these religions often claim superiority with resulting bloody and destructive wars between Protestant and Catholic Christians (Palatine Germany ethnic cleansing from 1619 to 1710 http://olivetreegenealogy.com/pal/overview.shtml) and between Shiite and Sunni Muslims and of course between different religious groups. Now President George W. Bush tries to evoke self defense in an invasion of Iraq and Afghanistan while claiming to be a Christian as have Western Christian leader done for 1500 years. Technologic preemptive defensive weapon development has also been tried. Dr. Richard Gatling invented his gun http://thebatteryguncompany.com/history.html and Albert Einstein encouraged President Roosevelt http://www.pbs.org/wnet/americanmasters/database/einstein_a.html to develop a nuclear weapon to help preempt fighting with lesser weapons with limited success. It may be better to treat: terrorists, violent fanatics of the East or West or Christian or Muslim or anarchist or fascist; as criminals if they harm or significantly threaten others and deal with them by laws, national and international, as appropriate for their crimes. With a truly nonbiased secure and private international security system this should be easily possible. If we had reduced our oil addiction as we had started to do in the 1970's and had failed to encourage extremist territorial Muslims [Osama Bin Laden] as we had in the 1980's to control the Soviet Union in Afghanistan and totalitarian Stalinists in Iraq [Saddam Hussein], we would be much more comfortable with the Middle East's peoples and Muslims. The Pew Research

Center documents our problems with other countries http:// pewresearch.org/reports/?ReportID=27. Defense of home territory real and virtual should be done first nonviolently and violently only as a last resort when all else fails. Information systems may help religions recognize the long-term needs of all peoples of the world, and to help limit institutional violence to only those situations that need immediate control of our primitive vertebrate physically harmful emotions.

Religion seeks to cover over and/or control our primitive genetic drives to help us avoid STI's (sexually transmitted infections), gluttony and violence. Muslims and conservative Christians do (and past generations of mainstream Christians have done) this by directly covering up the body and promoting denial of our basic genetic feelings or redirecting carnal love to spiritual love or agape. Given the AIDS epidemic we would benefit from prudent restricted intimate contacts. Fasting is still common and taken seriously by Muslims as it was in the past by Christians. Given our epidemic of obesity we likely should take fasting much more seriously. We might take the seven virtues of Christianity 1600 years ago more seriously http://en.wikipedia.org/wiki/Seven_virtues. The virtues emphasize compassion against the seven vices related to territoriality. The experience of confirmation may serve as a right of passage to help youth feel that they belong to the community committed to virtues. Frank Schaeffer in his book AWOL would have the USA require youths to spend 2 to 3 years in community or military service to help us regain the sense of community http://www.frankschaeffer.net/awol.html. Most religions emphasize the spiritual long-term goals and community needs over the individual's impulse of the moment. These impulses are hidden through our habits and culture to ease our social functioning. If we feel that the religious leaders give in to these hidden impulses often we may lose faith in this infrastructure of beliefs and move onto to a religion that more firmly helps its followers in meeting the daily temptations of our transient existence. Internationally we are closer to Muslin countries than to European countries in taking religion and God seriously. The Europeans trust more in governments and less in religion, while in the USA and in Muslim cultures we have more faith in religion and less in government http:// pewglobal.org/americaagainsttheworld/. In many ways the religious Muslims of the Middle East and the Christians of the USA are natural allies in combating short-term commercial interests that threaten our long-term goals. At present the USA commercial interests are too strongly imbedded in our culture and politics to allow us to make this international alliance to help us guide commercial corporations to work better for the long term interest of our species. A civil society needs this long-term community orientation to help its functions. In the USA our Constitution allows us to support those religions that best meet those goals. This freedom allows us to adapt so that in the future if we see the problem of excessive commercialization as being significant we may be able to control it.

Culture adapts more quickly with the changing consensus of populations of humans, unlike religious institutions with boards of life members with written texts and long memories that may only be changed slowly. Most cultures have accepted birth control with increased populations though religions often advise against it. A consensus recognizes that people often have sexual relations that are risky for STI's and unwanted pregnancies but are hard to resist due to our genetic drives. Most believe that adapting to the reality of this unwanted behavior is better than letting people suffer from some of the consequences that are untreatable. Religion may be right but in the present world with mass media and marketing of sweets and risqué fashion, impulses are emphasized over spirituality by most. With some rigid religious training and with aggressive marketing of the suggestive consumer products to our culture, we may suffer from religious and commercial extremism. The capitalist consumer market often benefits from ignoring religion and some religions benefit in the short term in blaming others for problems of their believers. This is a tragic conflict in that the conflict is inevitable when religion usually claims it is the truth and unchangeable and the commercial interests of the world stake their claim to the inalienable right in the West to market their products however questionable their social value for species survival. Truly the buyer must beware or in Latin "caveat emptor". We should encourage both sides to adapt to the best interests of the human race with a continuing non-violent discourse. Religion may need to adapt albeit slowly as an institution and commerce must recognize important environmental, genetic and religious values. Our ultimate goal of species survival with a diversity of people, their environments, and their attributes should be recognized by religion and our culture of commerce.

Cultures often emphasize the views of the majority and hide minority or outside opinions. This may reduce stress for the majority but if it happens to be wrong then it will lead to failure of the culture. Minority and outsider rights help inform the majority but do increase stress. Our constitutional system tries to balance these needs. The suppressing of local needs of populations has lead to the collapse of empires in the past and is threatening our commercial multinational western empire at the present. When empires become extended so much that the government is unable to respond or adapt to local needs of large numbers of people they collapse. The Roman Empire, The British Empire, and the Soviet Union found this out. The revolutionary founders of the USA were the inspiration for the Vietnamese and Cuban nationalists/communists and other groups seeking the ability to live in the way that they feel and know to be best for themselves and their own environment. Now multinational corporations seek to impose products on other cultures that may disrupt their feelings and health for short-term gains of profits without consideration of long-term disease and destruction from STI's, heart disease, cancer, lung disease, and economic dependence on fossil fuels. With better information and transparency within corporations hopefully they will adapt with the help of prudent boards, investors, and shareholders; else we may see a violent overthrow of over extended exploiting corporation CEO's and boards; or increasing terrorist attacks from the exploited, or those threatened by cultural and religious upheaval.

Specialists or technologists help to present information in their area of expertise. They may be corporate employees, bureaucrats, academics, consultants or a special interest advocate. The specialist will often emphasize his/her area of expertise and may use the information for power for him/herself or his/her employer or group. When high quality information is used without bias the specialists will keep corporations and governments functioning well by providing the correct information for efficient high quality products and services to the public. Groups or corporations with special interests may misuse them. Specialists are usually accurate on details but often try to hide the forest by having us concentrate on the trees to help their employer or favorite organization. In medicine, drug company representatives and pharmacy company hired medical consultants often emphasize the trivial minor advantages of their new drug without addressing a cost benefit analysis of their new drug compared with older less expensive (often generic) drugs.

Less subtle hiding occurs when corporations or governments do studies then hide the results that are unfavorable. With Vioxx positive studies were well-publicized and negative effects left unpublished or spun in a positive fashion. In the Department of the Interior the wilderness their experts studied land use but when they came up with a conclusion against the administration's policy it was ignored and kept from publication http://www.fs.fed.us/greatestgood/film/synopsis.shtml?sub2. Now some scientific journals are developing a policy to have all drug studies registered at their start and then keep track of the results in a public database so that negative effects as well as positive effects of drugs may be known (see Chapter 14 and Dr. Marcia Angell). For publicly traded companies on the stock markets the Sarbanes Oxley Act is attempting to make financial data on public corporations more accessible and understandable to help stockholders and boards of directors have better information to allow for better self governance http://en.wikipedia.org/wiki/Sarbanes_Oxley.

Data systems exist to help us build our information and form knowledge. Since the 1800's in the US we have had fairly extensive machine-readable information from the Census Bureau. They were early users of punch, Hollerith, or IBM cards http://en.wikipedia.org/wiki/Punched_card. Since the 1960's we have had birth, disease and death data in information systems in electronic form. These may help us evaluate social problems and plan to help people. Interpretation of raw data must be carefully done to obtain knowledge and wisdom. Huge numbers of deaths are caused by heart disease and cancer. Injuries cause much fewer deaths but they occur in younger people. When looking at the Years of Productive Life Lost (YPLL) injuries account for about a similar percent of YPLL as heart disease and cancer.

Data systems in the insurance and marketing are well advanced though hidden. Public health systems now lack the means to communicate or market healthy habits to consumers constantly bombarded by commercial messages to consume unhealthy products. Health insurance companies keep their data private to give them an advantage in negotiating with purchasers and health care providers. In the future Public Health Information Technology (PHIT) systems with payment decision support may make this information transparent and useful.

Feelings based on impressions and past experiences help direct our behavior. When health is valued at home and in the community and the person has positive health experiences, then health promotion and disease prevention is easier. Often health is associated with the denial of pleasurable experience or boring talks or programs or long waits at the doctor's office. Often eating junk food, drinking soda or alcohol, smoking, risk taking behavior, or sexual activity looks more desirable. Health and health care for the well may be tedious. Care for the ill should be emotionally supportive and free of blame. For public health we often are conflicted over caring for other people and protecting our own resources and property. With a good health care data system we may get all people cost effective care humanely and yet save more resources for society and ourselves.

We are often acculturated from childhood to suppress our feelings to avoid misbehaving at home and school. Guilt and shame often facilitate this. Often we develop bad habits when we connect with our feelings but hopefully we will be able to survive to a state of self-control without complete denial. The best control in our society is self-control from a well-educated and acculturated citizen. As Thomas Jefferson said, "The price of freedom is eternal vigilance."

With direct observation we may gain some basic information. Often what we see is dependent on our expectations. Some people when they see someone eating ice cream and enjoying it want to have some too but others may see someone getting too much sugar/fat/animal protein and too few vitamins. Some would taste the ice cream and enjoy but others would have concern for their health. For the calorie malnourished or underweight eating ice cream may be healthful. In some cultures and economic groups ice cream would be so expensive that its consumption would be a sign of a higher status or elite territory.

The ill effects poor health habits over the years are often hidden from the young and healthy. The ravages of diabetes, smoking and atherosclerosis with poor circulation are given much less attention than the partial cure for erectile dysfunction with a little pill advertised with billions of dollars. With the prevention of diabetes, smoking and hardening of the arteries, there would be much less erectile dysfunction with a lower cost and better outcome. With a more spiritual outlook we might care less about immediate gratifications.

For planning our future we need to know the reliability of our knowledge. Observing an association between some substance or behavior or environment, and health or disease gives some knowledge. Observing the association for many people and places at many different times increases the strength of the knowledge. If our understanding of basic science also suggests the association to be true then the association is more likely to predict the association to be true in the future and in many different circumstances. For the strongest predictive value it is best to observe what happens when we change the substance or behavior or environment for a large group of people and observe that their health improves or the disease goes away while a similar group of people without this change fails to improve in health or in the amount of disease. This is called an interventional study with a control group. When interventional studies with appropriate controls are done in many places with many different kinds of people at different times then it is unlikely that hidden unknown factors are effecting the association. This kind of association then would be expected to be important for similar people in similar places. These studies would make it safe to make changes in our culture to help improve health and decrease disease.

Let us now go on to address some important and common areas of health information. Mastering the information in these areas will help you and your neighbors feel better over your lifetimes while conserving your resources of energy, money and materials. For those of you who have had enough information or more than you want please go to Chapter 14, Information Overload: Too Much of a Good Thing. You may consult your physician for how to adjust your lifestyle to your body and community.

The rest of you may continue to browse the health information low calorie, low fat smorgasbord http://en.wikipedia.org/wiki/Smorgasbord.

CHAPTER 4
Sweets, Vitamin C, Obesity, Diabetes, and Scurvy

Our species' tendency to seek and eat sweets is partly responsible for 73,000 deaths in the US from diabetes http://www.cdc.gov/nchs/fastats/diabetes.htm and partly responsible for 690,000 heart disease deaths http://www.cdc.gov/nchs/fastats/heart.htm in 2002 in the USA. It may have been advantageous in our ancient prehistory to eat sweets when they where only found in the form of unrefined fruits or vegetables, but now this tendency predisposes us to succumb to market manipulation of our diets, tooth decay, obesity, diabetes and heart disease. Eating sweets hundreds of thousands of years ago also led us to lose our ability to make our own vitamin C. When we were getting all the vitamin C we needed in our diet this made us to be more efficient. We avoided wasting our energy on producing something in our bodies that we were already getting in abundance. When our culture changed our diet to eating less fresh foods and more refined sweets, then we became ill from the lack of vitamin C.

For most of us our genes direct us to eat sweets. This is information built into most of our bodies. From birth most of us have a genetic tendency to become content and seek to drink or eat more when our taste buds tell us we are eating something sweet. Eating sweet things does give us more energy or calories to grow and breed more. Sweets are often associated with romantic rituals. Often fruits that taste sweet give us Vitamin C. Our ancestor species ate large amounts of fruits and vegetables giving us large amounts of Vitamin C or ascorbic acid. At some point primates (the biologic family including us and monkeys) lost the ability to produce our own Vitamin C. Likely we were eating so much Vitamin C in our diet at that time hundreds of thousands of years ago that it made little difference in our survival. But starting about 4000 years ago humans began refining sugar. http://en.wikipedia. org/wiki/Sugar. First we extracted it from dates in the Middle East then later from beets and sugar cane. We devised a food that gave us calories and tasted good but lacked in the essential Vitamin C. The refined sugar also gives us tooth decay and too much gives us diabetes. Our biologic tendency to eat sweets that likely helped us survive and reproduce now may make us sick. Our food processing now has given us the sweetness in many foods but fails to give us the Vitamin C and with artificial sweeteners has even failed to give us calories. Sailors were the first large group to suffer Vitamin C deficiency or Scurvy when taking long voyages without fresh fruits and vegetables. A Spanish physician in Mexico wrote that citrus fruits would cure scurvy as early as 1592 (http://tidsskrift. kb.dk/centaurus/showtext.pl?ar_id=2&page=14). Sailors with scurvy often had food cravings. James Lind, a British naval surgeon, of the 1700's noted this and did a simple trial diet for sailors that showed that citrus juice prevented Scurvy. He published his study and conclusions in 1754 (http://www.bbc. co.uk/history/historic_figures/lind_james.shtml). The British Navy failed to order citrus fruit rations of lemon or lime for sailors until about 40 years later. Scurvy again attacks a large group of people in the late 1800's when food becomes more processed for large numbers of people.

Canning of fruits and vegetables, the use of processed foods, and the Pasteurization of milk help get rid of bacteria but they also get rid of Vitamin C. City dwellers, working in manufacturing, in the late 1800's mainly ate these processed foods. These foods were relatively cheap and would transport easily without spoiling. Refrigeration at home and in transportation was rare and expensive at that time. Often children are most affected since they require more Vitamin C due to their rapid growth. Breast milk for infants has Vitamin C in it if the mother is getting any Vitamin C. In the late 1800's many women were avoiding breast-feeding. This trend started in the upper classes with servants relegated to wet nursing or breast-feeding the infants. For the less affluent infants were fed pasteurized cow's milk or goat's milk or formulas. Scientists at that time only knew about proteins and calories but had failed to discover Vitamins until the early 1900's. The formulas for infants were developed scientifically but the science was deficient. The processed foods and formulas did help us avoid the common and often fatal bacterial diseases such as gastroenteritis from shigella and salmonella, and food born streptococcus, and they fit into the culture of manufacturing and science so we continued to use them.

The reasons for decreased breast-feeding in the 1800's, in contemporary America and increasingly around the world are unapparent due to their being suppressed by our taboos on sexuality and sensuality and in part by our unquestioning acceptance of the importance of short-term commercial success. Breast-feeding has a tradition going back to the start of us mammals. It also may be associated with intimate contacts and stimulation of uterine contractions with pleasurable feelings. In psychological testing images of breasts strongly attract the focus of our eyes. Often we must suppress this natural tendency by habits of looking away from breasts and cultural clothing habits that cover over distracting areas of the body. The same religious and cultural forces that would like to promote good health in infants also would like to prevent Sexually Transmitted Infections (STI's), sexual abuse of children, breast obsession, and marital instability. Breast-feeding promotion is a powder keg of unconscious forces. These forces may also help the species survival with better feeding in infancy and better attachment between mates to help the support of the mother and infant, therefore our conscious and subconscious must continually balance these forces with the help of religion and culture to benefit our families and children. See The Naked Ape and other writings by Desmond Morris http://www.desmond-morris.com/ for further observations on innate human tendencies shared with our primate ancestors.

Besides causing psychological stress from conflicts of the conscious and subconscious, breast-feeding often causes physical stress when sensitive skin has a baby firmly attached to it. Before the 1800's most fabric homespun or animal hides used for clothing were relatively rough so that they prepared the mother in part for some of the force that the baby would apply to the breast. Manufactured clothing of cotton that replaced the homespun and animal hides http://en.wikipedia.org/wiki/Undergarment was much softer; and soon replaced the rough and time consuming primitive clothing. The upper classes had even softer garments made of silk. In the 1940's and 50's nylon made the ultimate softness available to even the middle and lower classes.

The commercial interests lack any short-term benefits in promoting breast-feeding. Old style clothes may be expensive to make and are often uncomfortable. Formulas for infants make money for their manufacturers and allow mothers to avoid wrestling with many subconscious conflicts, pain when starting to breast feed, and difficulties in working or being in public places when breast feeding. Health insurance actually makes more money on illness than health so they lack any incentive to prevent disease. To promote good professional and public relations formula companies often do some promotion of breast-feeding but they lack the incentive to do a thorough and effective job. Physicians are mostly rewarded for doing procedures and seeing more patients. They lack any financial incentives to do more but do recommend breast-feeding to those who are interested in this healthy practice. Formulas now are much better than ever before due to advances in nutritional science, though we are unable to analyze what we fail to know about. Just recently we recognized a new nutrient docosahexaenoic acid (DHA) and put it into the latest formulas to help eye and brain development. It is possible there are other substances in breast milk and lacking in formula that might be discovered in the future. Some mothers need DHA supplements to get better levels in their milk and most babies need Vitamin D supplements when breast feeding for optimal health when breast feeding. Professor Colin Campbell of Cornell University believes that exposure of infants to cow's milk protein may promote cancer and autoimmune disease in children. His book presents the evidence: http://www.thechinastudy.com/ .

Some mothers with serious infections such as HIV (Human Immunodeficiency Virus) or Hepatitis C should avoid breast-feeding to prevent infecting their infant. Sometimes with breast-feeding babies will get more jaundice. Moms with high levels of organic mercury or other toxic chemicals or drugs should also avoid breast-feeding (link to reference on benefits and contraindications for breast feeding http://www.cdc.gov/breastfeeding/). Usually breast feeding is good for most infants and should be encouraged but present efforts fail to address adequately this complex issue due to little incentive to promote the many changes needed to want to and to be able to breast feed; and many incentives to formula feed. With PHIT (Public Health Information Technology) we should continually study any differences in formula feed infants and breast fed infants to help validate the quality of the different formulas and breast milk of mothers on different diets. The PHIT with confidential connections by e-mail and web sites might also be used to do targeted marketing of the best behaviors and diet for mothers, their babies and the supporting partner.

Many religious groups in the 1800's promoted eating traditional plant derived whole foods to purify the body. In the early 1900's it was discovered that guinea pigs, unlike most other animals, would get scurvy on a poor diet. In 1917 Scurvy was related to a deficiency to a vague substance called Vitamin C. In 1932 Albert Szent-Gyorgi isolated a crystal extract of Vitamin C from the rich source food of red pepper in his native Hungary. In 1933 Vitamin C was synthesized from xylose and then later glucose   www.gardenmosaics.cornell.edu/pgs/science/english/pdfs/peppers_teaching_tips.pdf. As is easily seen, we sometimes gather and use information from many sources to adapt to our environment. We also fail to use information such as food cravings in the sailors, the Spanish cures of scurvy by citrus fruit in 1592, and even the English report by Lind in 1754 took 40 years to change the standard practices of the British Navy. Our genetic tendency to eat sweets helps to get Vitamin C, but when we refine foods or are unable to eat our usual foods we get sick from the lack of Vitamin C, from diabetes, obesity and tooth decay. Physicians note that citrus fruits help cure and prevent Vitamin C deficiency or Scurvy in 1754. British bureaucrats after much delay put citrus fruits into the regular diet of sailors in 1794. Scientists eventually discover the substance Vitamin C or ascorbic acid in 1917. Bureaucrats put information on Vitamin C on food labels in the 1970's. Teachers educate children and professionals on the importance of Vitamin C in the 1920's. Some people adopt a religion or pattern of living to eat natural or whole foods to help get substances in foods that our bodies have evolved with in the 1800's. Some are just casual users of "health" foods or influenced by the advertising in our culture addressing our health concerns. We often desire or crave sweet food and that would direct us to Vitamin C in an ancient environment but in our present culture we might fail to get any Vitamin C from processed or chemically synthesized sweet foods. Our genetic tendencies tell us only that the behavior that gives us pleasure was once helpful in our survival and reproduction. It lacks information on the present new environmental elements. Genes that once gave us Vitamin C were lost because they failed to help us survive and reproduce in a food environment rich in Vitamin C. Bureaucrats in the British Navy or shipping companies may hide information on Scurvy to avoid the trouble of providing citrus fruit or juice to sailors. Manufacturers of food and fast food providers often avoid providing balanced meaningful nutritional information to help make selling profitable foods easier.

Since the 1960's manufacturer's recognized a market for low sugar drinks that still tasted sweet. This does help the diabetic or overweight person to decrease their sugar and calorie intake but has never been shown in clinical trials or for large numbers of people to help them reduce their weight. Some soft drink makers have done work with protein and vitamin containing drinks that may help people feel full while consuming less calories but yet still enough vitamins. As protein is more expensive than subsidized sugar and spoils easier, we will unlikely see much of these drinks until the public demands them. Professor Colin Campbell in www.thechinastudy.com/ points out that milk protein in excess increases cancer and perhaps heart disease. Soy or other plant protein drinks with 5% of the calories from plant protein might be better but it is generally best to eat the whole vegetables and/or fruits with the fiber to preserve the full nutritional benefits. Even drinks with some protein may contribute to obesity if they contain much fat or carbohydrate since it is easier to consume more calories in drinks than in food. Fat and carbohydrates would be needed to make the drinks more palatable.

Juice or fruit drinks are often proposed as an alternative to soda. Orange juice naturally contains vitamin C that is helpful. However large amounts of juice also contain large amounts of sugar that may also lead to obesity and tooth decay. Generally physicians recommend a daily consumption of no more than 8 ounces or 240mls of juice per day. Of course some juices such as apple juice fail to contain any vitamin C unless added to the juice in production. Many fruit drinks and even lemonade also fail to contain much vitamin C. Juice also lacks in much of beneficial fiber.

The United States of America still continues to subsidize sugar and corn syrup production despite our national obesity crisis and stated belief in free world trade. This continues to encourage junk food and soft drink manufacturers with increased profits, to load their products with the alluring easily marketable sweetness of sugar. Michael Pollan documents this in his book <u>The Omnivore's Dilemma</u> that he discussed on NPR (National Public Radio) http://www.npr.org/templates/story/story.php?storyId=5342514. We pay three times for this: once with subsidy payments, once with paying for the disease producing food, and once more with payments for the resultant diseases. Around 1900 in the United States we ate about 5 pounds of sugar per person and around 2000 we eat about 50 pounds of sugar per person and more of high fructose corn syrup http://www.illovo.co.za/worldofsugar/internationalSugarStats.htm. Given our commercial society and its emphasis on profits it is hard for the individual to avoid buying or receiving foods loaded with sugar.

Past approaches to healthy living and intervention studies have failed to decrease obesity for most people with relatively simple interventions http://www.nytimes.com/2006/02/14/health/14fat.html?ex=1140584400&en=0d2fb06cc2a24d8e&ei=5070&emc=eta1 . Simply eating simple foods and whole grains as Rev. Sylvester Graham recommended or chewing well a low protein diet as Horace Fletcher advocated about 100 years ago failed to guarantee a lean figure. Long before Dr Robert C. Atkins, Jean Anthelme Brillat-Savarin recommended a low carbohydrate diet to promote health with only modest success. Many diet plans work for some or for some short time periods but long-term obesity control is often hard to obtain. Even with overweight children who have less ingrained habits change is often hard to achieve http://www.nytimes.com/2006/02/12/weekinreview/12kolata.html?ex=1140411600&en=c74ee02f726ab400&ei=5070&emc=eta1 . Effective nutrition and exercise education and healthier choices in school menus failed to make any impact on obesity in intervention trials in the 1990's. http://www.ncbi.nlm.nih.gov/entrez/query.

fcgi?cmd=Retrieve&db=pubmed&dopt=Abstract&list_uids=14594792&query_hl=3&itool=pubmed_docsum

The researchers suggest community wide interventions. Or perhaps kids and adults are smarter than we give them credit for. Perhaps kids in our tumultuous world with street crime and centralized food supply that is always under threat from natural or man-made disasters / terrorist attacks/ wars/ energy crises know in their subconscious the advantage of carrying extra energy supplies with them. These maybe kids that tend to get anxious or are naturally cautious. Perhaps we need to increase their security with decentralizing supplies, creating community support/ storage capacity for food and energy and safe and rewarding ways to exercise and produce or at least save on usable energy at the same time. Simply safe walkways, playgrounds, community gardens, local farms, and human powered vehicles on safe pathways (bicycles/tricycles with all weather and easy storage capacity) may help.

We could use new more complex interventional studies with PHIT to see what reducing sugar content in foods, increasing exercise, and changing the community environment would do for most people. Would they get negative feelings or anxious or just get a weight more appropriate for their size? Would they have less intimate contacts or fewer children or more divorces? Would they be more tired or less tired? Would people feel threatened by lack of privacy in community programs? Past experiences with famines during World War II have shown diabetes rates to go down but is it possible in our open society with commercial distractions to self-impose fasting or self-deprivation? Would large numbers of representative people consent to using their grocery store purchases and credit card food purchases be tracked? Would they allow their refrigerators and cupboards to be Internet linked to read the user's bar code identifier and bar code the food used? How would diet changes affect activity, exercise, and home air temperature changes? Would people use hydrogen or electricity generating exercise equipment? Would people use human powered weather protected vehicles or just walk more to nearby locations? Would people invest in community safety, exercise availability, and decentralized food and energy supplies? Would people allow their doctor's weight loss program's records on weight, height, environment and behavior to be used to help study this important issue? If so we could gain some insight into what kind of diet, exercise and community changes might help most people.

CHAPTER 5
Tobacco: A Stimulus to the Modern Economy with Bad Side Effects

Tobacco entered into common use in European American culture in the 1500's when the Spanish discovered and marketed a strain of tobacco that could be easily smoked in pipes or inhaled as snuff. The native Americans or as Columbus called them the "Indians" did have tobacco perhaps thousands of years before the Spanish connected with them but most of it was very bitter and irritating when smoked. It was fine for ceremonial purposes but not an every day substance in the Americas before Columbus and his Spanish colleagues got there. The Spanish found a particular strain or cultivar of tobacco that could enjoyably be smoked or used for snuff and then grew it on the Island of Hispaniola (now Haiti and the Dominican Republic). From 1500 to 1600 their exports to Europe of tobacco earned them more wealth than all the gold they captured and mined from the New World. To break the tobacco monopoly of the Spanish an Englishman John Rolfe in 1612 obtained some plants from the Caribbean then brought them to the English Colony of Virginia to grow. To his pleasant surprise the tobacco plants did well in Virginia and tobacco became more affordable and accessible for Americans, Europeans and eventually others: http://www.apva.org/history/jrolfe.html. John Rolfe in 1614 married the Indian Princess Pocahontas or Motoaka http://www.powhatan.org/pocc.html .

She was kidnapped in 1612 and held captive for ransom in Jamestown by the English until she married. She was converted to Christianity and renamed Rebecca. John Rolfe and Rebecca had a son Thomas: http://www.apva.org/history/pocahont.html. Rebecca died in 1617 in England where she had visited with John Rolfe and helped raise money and interest in the Virginia Company. She died of a respiratory illness that was likely tuberculosis. Her husband, son and his descendents survived to continue with others the Virginia tobacco industry that eventually helped to pleasantly stimulate many and to bring about many heart attack, cancer and lung disease deaths.

Tobacco now causes about one in five deaths or 440,000 deaths per year in the United States. The CDC says it is the largest cause of preventable deaths in our country:
http://www.cdc.gov/tobacco/factsheets/Tobacco_Related_ Mortality_factsheet.htm . Tobacco use in pipes starting in the 1500's to 1600's, increases lip and mouth cancer risk. Snuff is most popular in the 1700's with increased risk of nasal cancer noted. Cigars and chewing tobacco are most popular in the 1800's with increased risk of mouth cancer. Cigarettes start to be mass produced in the late 1800's and are given to troops in World War I. Lung cancer and heart attack rates rise with the increased use of cigarettes:
http://www.tobacco.org/resources/history/Tobacco_ History.html . In the 1950 Ernst Wynder, MD published a large case control study using a mathematically sound case control analysis that showed smoking cigarettes was strongly linked to bronchiogenic cancer http://www.cdc.gov/mmwr/ preview/mmwrhtml/mm4843bx.htm and
http://tc.bmjjournals.com/cgi/content/full/8/4/444. About 7,000 studies confirmed the link and on January 11, 1964,

Luther L. Terry, M.D., Surgeon General of the U.S. Public Health Service, released the report of the Surgeon General's Advisory Committee on Smoking and Health. http://www.cdc. gov/tobacco/sgr/sgr_1989/1989SGRIntro.htm

The Report confirmed that cigarette smoking is a definite risk for lung cancer and a likely risk for many other diseases. We might surmise that you would have to be crazy to smoke. Recent studies suggest that it helps. In the February 4, 2006 Journal of the American Medical Association (JAMA), a news article reports that much higher portions of people with schizophrenia and Attention Deficit Disorder (ADD) smoke than portions of people without mental disabilities.

Smoking seems to help people cope with modern industrial life at least in the short run. Nicotine the main active ingredient in cigarettes acts as a stimulant to help concentration in people with ADD and helps normalize brain function in people with schizophrenia http://www.nida.nih.gov/NIDA_notes/ NNvol20N2/NIDA.html. ADD and schizophrenia have genetic components that may make some people more susceptible to nicotine addiction than others. Smoking cigarettes is associated with blue-collar mass production or assembly line workers who often must pay attention to repetitive mind numbing tasks. Cigarettes with their nicotine likely help the worker perform better and safer on the immediate tasks. As countries industrialize smoking becomes much more common as mass manufacturing increasing availability and assembly lines increasing desirability. China now has increasing smoking rates and will have increasing lung cancer and heart disease rates in 10 to 20 years as we had 50 years ago. The problems with cigarettes come from the tobacco tars that produce carcinogens or cancer causing substances and lung irritants when burned and the carbon monoxide from the burning that causes hardening of the arteries. Presently we use nicotine patches or gum (or inhalers in research studies) to help people stop smoking but their convenience, price and availability make them less usable than cigarettes. http://www.sciencedaily.com/releases/2003/05/030530081654.htm

http://bmj.bmjjournals.com/cgi/content/full/321/7257/329

Coffee or colas or other caffeinated drinks also are used as stimulants with more safety. Often sugar consumption is increased with these drinks with the side effects of obesity, tooth decay and heart clogging fats or lipids but if taken without sugar they are fairly safe. Some people do get rapid heart rates with caffeine and should avoid it but else it seems quite safe. Prescribed stimulants such as dexamphetamines and methylphenidates do help ADD but are controlled substances that may cost $45 to $60 per month and require a doctor's supervision. For attention problems and also anxiety and/or depression tricyclic antidepressants such as amitriptyline or imipramine may help. Anxiety controlling bupropion may help some especially during the nicotine withdrawal stage. SSRI's (selective serotonin reuptake inhibitor) such as fluoxetine (Prozac) may also help ADD, depression and anxiety. Street drugs may also have stimulant effects but are unreliable in contents and strength and have severe legal consequences with purchase or possession. Anything injectable and shared nose straws may give the user HIV (Human Immunodeficiency Virus or AIDS virus) or Hepatitis C virus infections unless extreme caution is taken with the sterility of the injections and works. Instead of medicating workers some manufacturers such as Volvo have tried to make the process more interesting and rewarding psychologically. They try to give workers different tasks or modules to accomplish with other team or work group members to give them more of a challenge to their intelligence and sense of an accomplishment for completing a larger part of the product or the complete product if possible. This approach is now rare and its health affects little studied.

In retrospect it is amazing that we have made the rapid transition (in terms of genetic and religious time frames) from an agricultural based economy to an industrial based economy with the stress based diseases of depression and anxiety only severely affecting 10% of the population at some time in their life http://www.cdc.gov/mentalhealth/data.htm. In only 6 generations we have radically changed the way we live and are still adapting in culture and religion and are only just starting to adapt genetically. The 440,000 deaths from tobacco use per year occurring in mid to later life is part of the price we pay for changing how we live. Even if we adapt to or cure all current disease we will inevitably produce new diseases as we change the way we live. Disease is just a maladaptation to our way of life and environment. With so much of knowledge hidden from us we are bound to make mistakes when we change how we live based just on what we know. Gradual change based on our best current knowledge and with close observations of what happens with change is best. Starting with small groups or research studies is best. Improving our health and social information technology should enable us to continuously and efficiently study what happens as we change our habits, diet, environment, economy and our health care.

CHAPTER 6
Cholesterol: a Study in Medical Ignorance

In the 1950's Ancel Keys saw a clear connection between high cholesterol in the diet and in the blood; and coronary artery heart disease. He was right in part but it is rare that any simple statement regarding complex phenomena is completely true. In the late 1800's and early 1900's tuberculosis and infectious disease were the major killers. Coronary heart disease though had started in the upper classes in the late 1800's and was affecting the middle and some of the lower class by the 1950's. Before this time coronary heart disease was rare. The coronaries are the arteries that carry oxygen to the heart muscle. If they get blocked then we may feel pressure like chest pain and within a ½ hour the heart muscle will start to get damaged. Previously people might have had Rheumatic Heart Disease due to recurrent Group A Streptococcal infections. Through the work of Ancel Keys and many other investigators from around the world in studying cholesterol and saturated fat levels in the diet, blood levels of cholesterol and the incidence of coronary heart disease in 7 countries we thought that eating a high cholesterol and/or high saturated fat diet would increase the risk of coronary heart disease and heart attacks http://www.ncbi.nlm.nih.gov/entrez/query.fcgi?cmd=Retrieve&db=pubmed&dopt=Abstract&list_uids=7586324&query_hl=6&itool=pubmed_docsum and http://www.washingtonpost.com/wp-dyn/articles/A7213-2004Nov23.html.

Cholesterol is found in egg yolks, butter, milk fat, and in meats. Saturated fat is the hard fat found in meats, in butter, and milk fat. Blood or serum cholesterol generally goes up as the amount of cholesterol and saturated fat in the diet goes up. There is also a large amount of genetic variation in the amount of cholesterol that each person produces regardless of diet consumed. In the late 1800's the upper classes were eating more meat and butter that were relatively expensive then. The wealthy over weight banker or other sedentary affluent middle age male became victims of their new life style. The studies in the late 1950's showed that males in the United States who had diets high in cholesterol and saturated fat were at much higher risk than males with low cholesterol and low saturated fat diets in Mediterranean countries. In the early 1960's the Framingham studies showed that individuals with high serum cholesterol had a much greater chance of heart attacks and coronary heart disease than individual with average or low serum cholesterols http://www.nhlbi.nih.gov/about/framingham/timeline.htm. Framingham also helped link smoking to heart attacks. Ancel Keys went on to live near Naples, Italy and eat a Mediterranean diet with vegetables especially beans, fruits, and some olive oil; and lived to be a 100 years old in pretty good shape until he was 97.

Many of the rest of us went on to eat French fries, low fat high sugar ice cream, fried chicken, and potatoes with hard margarine and were still dying of heart disease. In 2002 697,000 people in the United States died of heart disease http://www.cdc.gov/nchs/fastats/heart.htm. Cholesterol and saturated fat in our diet is just a part of the problem. In the mid 1960's we were suffering from medical ignorance of what dietary and lifestyle factors, beyond dietary cholesterol and saturated fat, make a difference to our heart health. We even failed to know that we did not know other important dietary factors for heart health. Even worse we thought we knew everything. So we went right ahead to eliminating or decreasing cholesterol and saturated fat from our diet often replacing them with things that were just about as bad: added refined sugar and hydrogenated vegetable oil with trans-saturated fatty acids. We now know that added sugar and even carbohydrates such as bread without fiber will increase our blood sugar levels and thereby increase our own insulin. When we produce more insulin we then produce more of the bad fats in our blood stream such as LDL's or low-density lipoproteins and triglycerides that clog our coronary and other arteries. If we are unable to produce more insulin then we get diabetes that causes our tiny blood vessels or capillaries to clog and results in heart, eye, nerve, and kidney disease. If we eat more sugars or carbohydrates or starches we get excessive fat in our bellies or abdomen that may increase our blood pressure. The trans-saturated fats increase the blockage in our arteries by fats. Trans-saturated fats in vegetable shortening or hard margarine are often found in deep fried foods and baked goods. We also eliminated or reduced from our diet egg yolks, which are a major inexpensive and safe source of DHA (docosahexaenoic acid). Egg yolks also have much cholesterol but with reduced calories and much oat bran in our diet we might avoid increasing our blood cholesterol levels even if we ate some eggs. DHA helps our blood vessels be more flexible, helps our eyes, helps our memory and decreases inflammation. DHA also is present in fish and fish oil. DHA may also be derived from oils in walnuts and flaxseed. Because of mercury in fish we should avoid eating tuna fish or swordfish or other large fish more than once a week http://www.cfsan.fda.gov/~dms/admehg3.html .

Trans-saturated fats or infectious disease such as mycoplasma or Chlamydia TWAR may cause inflammation in our arteries. The information about how refined sugar, trans-saturated fatty acids and DHA deficiency make our coronary arteries and hearts worse was unavailable in the mid 1960's http://www.fda.gov/fdac/features/2003/503_fats.html .

Could we have avoided these errors? Yes by trying controlled double blind intervention trials. These are studies where one group has an active intervention and another similar group has a different probably inactive intervention, then observers who lack any knowledge of the interventions used on the particular subjects notes the outcomes. It is called double blinded because the subjects and the observers are both blind to the intervention used on the individuals. Someone who matches the interventions to the outcomes analyzes the results objectively. To test if we really know how things work we must intervene based on our best knowledge then observe to see if the expected results happen. In the mid 1960's most physicians and technicians or bureaucrats thought we knew enough to have everyone change their lifestyle based on their knowledge at the time. Sure hundreds of thousands of USA residents were dying of heart disease and we would all feel bad if we denied possibly beneficial treatments or diet changes from people with looming mortal threats. Though if we were cynical, cautious, or humble enough we may have appreciated that our possibly beneficial interventions might actually been harmful and we would have been correct in part. Medical ignorance is a serious matter http://www.ignorance.medicine.arizona.edu/index.html.

Vitamin E supplementation also demonstrated the flaw in assuming a simple new intervention to be harmless. People with Vitamin E levels above normal were found to have better hearts. Vitamin E is an antioxidant safe in the short run in large doses so why not try it in large amounts with anyone at risk for heart disease? Of course you are thinking to yourself "Why not indeed, because it could be harmful!" Which it was as shown in controlled intervention trials in the past 2 years demonstrating increased heart related disease in study subjects using large amounts of Vitamin E for sick patients http://www.ncbi.nlm.nih.gov/entrez/query.fcgi?cmd=Retrieve&db=pubmed&dopt=Abstract&list_uids=16087144&query_hl=1&itool=pubmed_docsum and http://www.ncbi.nlm.nih.gov/entrez/query.fcgi?cmd=Retrieve&db=pubmed&dopt=Abstract&list_uids=15753154&query_hl=1&itool=pubmed_DocSum. Despite this hundreds of websites offer to sell you Vitamin E to supposedly decrease your risk of heart disease http://www.nlm.nih.gov/medlineplus/druginfo/natural/patient-vitamin-e.html. In July 2006 The CSPI (Center for Science in the Public Interest) in their nutrition newsletter said the consumption of Vitamin E did decrease 25% in the past year. Perhaps the consumer is informed.

Beyond the overconfidence, excessive ego strength, and deficiency of cynicism there was also problems with the logistics and expense of carrying out a large-scale long-term cultural and medical intervention trial. Without basic electronic medical records, performing medical or lifestyle intervention trials often is prohibitively expensive. If you have a drug that is patented and capable of generating a large income then separate medical care and data systems may be created to document its usefulness. All the egg industry had was chicken feed, humility and patience. An intervention trial was eventually started in the 1970's with multiple risks addressed and with a comparison with standard care as the control intervention- the Multiple Risk Factor Intervention Trial or

MRFIT Study http://www.nhlbi.nih.gov/resources/deca/ descriptions/mrfit.htm . Its interventions for blood pressure, cholesterol/diet and activity did produce a 5 to 10% decrease in heart disease compared with standard medical care. For the expense of the interventions this was only a marginal effect, likely due to the many important factors in heart disease unknown at the time including the need to markedly reduce animal fat and protein to maximally benefit our hearts. Colin Campbell says that diet intervention should eliminate all animal protein/fat, and refined sugars to be most effective http://www.thechinastudy.com/. In MRFIT the intervention group and the control group had diets that were very similar from his international prospective. In China many rural areas have people with cholesterol levels in the 80's. In MRFIT and even now we often settle for levels below 200. Michael Pollan points out that a basic problem with being an omnivore such we humans are is that we have so many choices to make in eating http://www.npr.org/templates/story/ story.php?storyId=5342514. In the future if we develop our health information technology infrastructure we may more easily evaluate associations of habits such as diets high in fiber or DHA and/or low in animal protein and fat, exercise, meditation, or inflammation measured by c reactive protein or high sedimentation rates, with heart disease and then design and evaluate interventions based on these observations. This is the never ending observe, intervene, evaluate intervention and observe again etc. cycle. Using PHIT (public health information technology) we would be able to pay low marginal costs for studies of simple inexpensive interventions that might be very effective. We might even reincarnate MRFIT into the new century as MRPHIT.

Until we get all the results of future studies on how best to prevent disease, what should a prudent adult do to prevent heart and other diseases now? For most people a low salt, low sugar, low saturated fat, high oat and wheat fiber, 5 servings of fruits and vegetables per day, some nuts, Vitamin D 500 units per day, Vitamin E 50 to 100 units per week, and DHA 100 mg per day diet; with minimal abdominal or belly fat, non-smoking, ½ to 1 glass of wine per week for men, some low sugar chocolate, and regular exercise of ½ hour of more 3 times a week would help. Chocolate and wine, just as fruits and vegetables, have key chemicals or bioflavinoids that are good for our heart and body. Wine at more than 1 glass a week seems to increase breast cancer risk for women. Lowering animal protein consumption to 5% or less of our calorie intake would also likely help. Now most people in the USA get about 20 to 30% of their calories from animal protein. Colin Campbell would simply suggest just use only whole plant based foods such as whole grains, legumes, dark greens, nuts, seeds and fruits http://www.thechinastudy.com/. For people living more than 30 degrees north or south of the equator should take Vitamin D in the winter. People with dark skin or those staying indoors most of the time also need Vitamin D. People avoiding animal protein completely should take Vitamin B12 oral supplements or nutritional brewer's yeast. Correctly chosen whole plant based foods would give you Vitamin E in whole grains and DHA precursors in walnuts and flaxseed. See a doctor with knowledge in nutrition and/or nutritionist to more finely adjust your lifestyle to your genetics and environment. For many now, medications to lower blood pressure and cholesterol often do help prevent heart and stroke problems when other interventions fail. Cholesterol lowering medications may cause muscle problems. Blood pressure lowering medications may cause fatigue or electrolyte problems. Extremes of any single intervention seem tempting but often fail. Much exercise and a diet high in saturated fat and sugar may still give coronary artery disease. A starvation diet would eventually give heart disease from protein deficiency or malnutrition, though would give you cleaner arteries. This is part of the art of living and of medicine to design a way to live that is satisfying and sustainable. Many now call for Evidence Based Medicine but often "The logic is uncertain" as Mr. Spock the Vulcan from Star Trek would say. Dr. Spock would say to go vegan or vegetarian without eggs or dairy products http://www.cnn.com/HEALTH/9806/20/dr.spock/index.html . In the future a PHIT with inexpensive genetic testing information might help us determine better what environment, diet, medication, treatment or combination thereof is best for certain key genetic types but with 30,000 genes and millions of combinations much art will still be left to us and our doctors. Colin Campbell does point to the numerous studies of ethnic groups of people who have low heart disease, cancer and autoimmune diseases in their home territory and then get these diseases when they move to a developed country and eat the common high animal protein diet of that developed country http://www.thechinastudy.com/. Eating the whole food plant based diet is likely best for most people despite genetic variations and hopefully our future efficient, private and secure information systems will prove it or disprove it and detect any unforeseen problems and/or improvements with this dramatic change in our diet.

CHAPTER 7
Sexually Transmitted Infections: Taboo for Two

All of you that have gone to the medical ignorance website already know that another common cause of medical ignorance is taboo or denial. Often our subconscious, our culture or both forbid us to even think about such things http://www.ignorance.medicine.arizona.edu/index.html Fortunately for our survival and unfortunately for your subconscious and immediate pleasure potential, public health and other hard-nosed physicians and religious leaders are ready to spoil your fun for your and our own good. Culture stars sometimes join in prevention programs when immediate risks of sexual contacts are great but in the commercial West they often cheerlead for immediate gratification at least in fantasies. Hopefully thinking about infectious disease and psychological risks of close or intimate contacts will at least save you some of the stress of being unable to decide what to do in a pressure situation. This is nothing new. For at least 3,000 years we have been trying to control Sexually Transmitted Infections (STI's) by morality and laws. By observing our primate relatives and isolated cultures that live isolated from others in small groups we believe that ancient prehistoric humans often had sexual contacts with multiple partners. Dominant males in the small groups often would protect their female partners from contacts with other males through a hierarchy enforced by violent action as needed. This behavior is called mate guarding. Females often would mate with many males when ovulating (and evading mate guarding) due to hormonal effects promoting fertilization of the egg just released from the ovary into the fallopian tubes. Fertilization of the egg would be determined by sperm competition among the sperm donors who got their sperm into the vagina. Males with more and faster sperm would be favored to have genetic progeny. In simple societies without exposure to germs and where mates were in close contact this worked adequately. When males went the fields to work, or to distant cities for trading this system caused spread of STI's and created anxiety. In small groups women might get support for their children from relatives or other group members. In a city or large village the support might be lacking. About 3000 years ago civil and religious laws, such as the 10 Commandments evolved to provide protection in the new complex environment. With marriage the mates committed to each other and the adults committed to feed, shelter and raise the children created within the marriage. This relieved the male of some mate guarding anxiety and the need to continually fight off rival males, and guaranteed the women and children the rights of support. Territory groups, city states or nations would take on mate guarding responsibilities and assistance in promoting support of children in return for taxes and loyalty to the political unit. Of course our genetic tendencies to seek and enjoy sex are still there to produce stress between our subconscious and conscious at times. Religion and culture sometimes battle over and sometimes cooperate on how to handle this intrinsic conflict.

Our present state of affairs favors the institution of marriage and the suppression of sexually desires outside of long-term monogamous relationships. Close warm moist contacts have always been a great way to pass germs. When most people lived in small groups and had few contacts with outsiders of any kind, germs would travel slowly and would be limited to small geographic areas. With large cities and rapid worldwide transportation the HIV (Human Immunodeficiency Virus) spread from African cities to Europe and the United States within months in 1981. As early as 1959 it existed in rural African areas where it was originally a virus in chimpanzees or other animals that mutated into a human borne virus http://fohn. net/history-of-aids/. As with many STI's and other contagious diseases, HIV spreads before the person has any signs of illness. AIDS (Acquired Immunodeficiency Disease Syndrome) often takes 6 months or more to develop after the initial infection with HIV. For at least a few months HIV infected people are contagious without any symptoms. Simply staying away from anyone who is sick is inadequate to prevent AIDS or HIV infection or most other infectious diseases. In the United States of America (USA) and Europe we are able to control the HIV infection and get rid of AIDS by taking medications 2 or more times a day, and getting frequent medical supervision that is expensive. For most of these patients HIV is only temporarily suppressed and AIDS will start up anytime the medication is discontinued. In North America in 2005 about 30,000 people died of AIDS http://www.unaids.org/en/Regions_Countries/default.asp . In areas of the world without such medical resources, HIV quickly progresses to AIDS and the patient dies within 1 to 2 years. In 2005 in sub Saharan Africa 2.4 million people died of AIDS. Some of these deaths in Africa may be delayed with simple less expensive medications for infections that complicate AIDS such as tuberculosis, malaria, and pneumocystis carinii pneumonia (PCP). Now HIV is present around the world with over 15% of people in Southern Africa infected and about 0.5 to 1% of North Americans infected http://www.childinfo.org/eddb/hiv_aids/index.htm . In 2007 USA help to Africa for better treatment of AIDS is helping with purchase and distribution of medications http://www.pbs.org/wgbh/pages/frontline/aids/etc/links.html. Even if we could cure AIDS, get rid of HIV with medication (not possible now), and prevent HIV infection with a safe and effective vaccine (not possible in the foreseeable future), we still should avoid close, warm and wet contacts with multiple partners.

Once one germ is controlled another will soon take its place. Before HIV and AIDS spread throughout the world the bacterium Treponema pallidum and the disease Syphilis kept millions in fear. In the 1950's we were able to control this disease with penicillin http://en.wikipedia.org/wiki/Syphilis#History . If untreated, Syphilis causes long term damage to the heart and brains that may be debilitating or fatal and may damage infants born to infected mothers. It is likely that Treponema pallidum came from a less harmful bacterium that existed some in Europe or the Caribbean. Columbus and his crew picked up the newly mutated bacteria and quickly spread it by sexual and perhaps skin infections among their New World and Old World sexual and intimate contacts. By 1530 it was common in both Europe and the Americas. It is likely that other germs exist in mild forms in our own or other species that may mutate and spread quickly if given the chance by our sexual, close, or blood contact. Given the past history of germs jumping species we should also avoid close contacts with blood or body fluids even with other species. In the 1950's penicillin also was able to control the bacterium Neisseria gonorrhea or Gonorrhea that had been around for a few thousand years http://www.cdc.gov/std/Gonorrhea/ . This was a fairly common cause of disease but usually not fatal. Now Gonorrhea requires newer or more expensive antibiotics for treatment but in the 1950's it also became less of a problem with the use of penicillin. In combination with birth control pill availability and IV drug abuse the stage was set for a new epidemic STI HIV that was also contagious through blood as is Syphilis. If condoms were still used, contacts were limited, and blood contamination avoided, HIV would have had a much less damaging impact.

The World Wide Web with multimedia has served people with sexual interests. Much too often this was used to encourage deviant behavior that may have lead to disease or abuse of children. Some electronic dating has lead to abusive relationships due to unrealistic expectations. The first use of video conferencing seemed to be dominated by voyeurs and exhibitionists. As long as they were consenting adults this is much better than doing it in public without consent. In the future with biofeedback and surgical manipulation capabilities over the Internet virtual contact might be made with less risk for biologic germs and abusive or violent relationships or as in the film <u>AI</u> (Artificial Intelligence <u>http://en.wikipedia. org/wiki/A.I. %28film%29</u>) robots might eventually serve as prostitutes. This would eliminate biologic germ risks if done properly and prevent human exploitation but still would be distracting and addictive for humans. Abstinence when possible would be less wasteful of resources. With social encouragement and nutritional fasting from sugar and/or animal protein abstinence might be more popular. Encouraging abstinence for singles, marriage for partners, and clean non-exploitive orgasms for those that are unable to abstain or stay in a monogamous relationship will be a challenge at the new frontier for morality, ethics, and religion.

In order to treat and control current STI's and detect new STI's we need a PHIT (Public Health Information System) that is private and secure in real time. To be sure all people with STI disease get treated and to prevent spread to others strict confidentiality must be insured in such a sensitive area with risks of violent mate guarding, shame, embarrassment, and guilt. The PHIT may also be used to prevent, through vaccination registries and reminders, some STI's such as Hepatitis B and the human papillomavirus that causes cervical and uterine cancer. In STI clinics and other confidential areas patients should be given the option of using an assumed name though all must use a unique identifying number that might just be kept on a smart card with a photo but without a name. The Electronic Health Record and the PHIT would know the patient's true identity but health care providers would only know as much as the patient chooses them to know. The patient by concealing parts of their health information would assume liability for any errors caused by an incomplete medical and health record. The patient might allow through an advance directive or health care proxy the disclosure of information if they were seriously ill or unconscious or they may choose that they would rather die than have a breech of confidentiality. Once the patient has made the choice the information would be entered on the PHIT for use as directed at medical offices, clinics, emergency care and hospitals. The linked PHIT information would be used to notify and if needed to treat contacts in a confidential and private manner to prevent further spread of disease. The PHIT would monitor for new STI's, new resistant strains of STI's, and the effects of diet, exercise, and multimedia on sexual behavior, exploitive behavior and STI's. In matters of public danger or terrorism or national security or serious criminal investigation with court ordered warrants such information might be used on a strict need to know basis by public officials for health and safety only. Analysis of linked records, without any identifying information, for epidemiological and scientific studies should be encouraged rather than be discouraged as is now the case with many of the current HIPPA regulations http://www.cms.hhs.gov/HIPAAGenInfo/01 Overview.asp.

CHAPTER 8
Preventing Injuries: Searching for Our Best Niche

Often when we think of injuries we are perplexed as to why they happen. We often called them accidents because they seemed to lack any cause. The basic reasons for them are so fundamental that they just reside in our subconscious often hidden from rational consideration, though widely dealt with in the arts. Usually injuries occur as we compete for favorable environmental resources or we venture into hostile environments to gain untapped resources. In nutrient rich coastal waters our fish vertebrate ancestors would be eaten by other species or fight with other members of their own species for territory to be able to obtain the resources needed to mate and support their offspring. Eventually fins evolved into legs and new the vertebrates moved onto land or God put some species there. In this hostile environment drying out, overheating, overcooling, or surf damage could be fatal. Our primate ancestors or fellow creations took to the trees to avoid terrestrial predators and gain new food sources though suffered the new injuries of tree falls. To avoid competition with other species members for limited prime property we may spread out across the earth into relatively hostile areas with excess cold, heat altitude, dryness, or water. With competition we may fight others for environments rich with natural resources and comfortable to live in. Through evolutionary prehistory and our recent known history we must adapt to find the best way to survive and flourish: to stake our claims to prized property and defend it, or to brave the hazards of a new territory and gain its resources. Often we vertebrates may fight for mates directly or indirectly by building and protecting resource rich nest sites or territories. Gaining the mate and/ or guarding the mate may entail some combat, though much less now than in our precivilized past. This explains much of jealousy, lover's quarrels, male/ female rivalry, gang violence, ethnic "cleansing", and racial tension. In the antebellum South of the USA many Africans bore children with European genes as part of the institutionalized subjugation of the Africans. After the Civil War black men were lynched for just thinking or acting in anyway like they might mate with Europeans as part of the great fear of possible mate infidelity brought on by the sudden cultural change. In the Oneida Community, allowing the elderly board of governors to determine who the mate pairs should be; institutionalized mate guarding. They often chose male board members as being the ones to mate with the most desirable young female Community members. They justified this on the basis of the new science of eugenics. The Community then lost its young males who ventured into new environments to get better resources and mate choices. The Community then broke up http://libwww.syr.edu/digital/ guides/o/OneidaCommunityCollection/. Hitler later took up eugenics from America and used it to institutionalize his racial mate-guarding program http://www.frontpagemag.com/ Articles/ReadArticle.asp?ID=10004. Hitler concentrated on intraspecies violence and actually disliked interspecies violence. He emphasized violent mate guarding for his genetic group but often avoided violence against other species http://en.wikipedia. org/wiki/Vegetarianism_of_Adolf_Hitler.

Now let's look at our huge numbers of young and some old people that die from injuries in the United States of America (USA) and at how we may adapt to decrease the numbers.

In the USA in 2002 injuries caused 161,269 deaths. Of these 106,742 were unintentional or related to humans going into hostile environments and 49,293 due to intraspecies violence http://www.cdc.gov/nchs/fastats/injury.htm. The hostile environment with the largest single contribution to unintentional deaths is the highway with 44,065 deaths in that year. We venture into this hostile environment to become more productive (with work and trade) thus getting more resources for our families and social groups; and we increase our possibilities for mating with easy travel. As with much technology that we use to extend into new environments we tend to have less risk per person as we adapt to using the technology better. Engineers offer safe choices such as seat belts, car seats, booster seats, and traffic control signals (stop lights); and better when possible they build the safety into their product with safer dash boards, air bags, crumple zones, divided highways and controlled access to further eliminate human judgment errors http://www.cdc.gov/health/motor.htm. In 1930 we had about 44,000 deaths from Motor Vehicle-related Injuries (MVI's) with much fewer drivers, people and automobiles. Our rate of deaths from MVI's per 100,000 people in 1950 was 24.6 and was down to 15.7 in 2002 http://www.cdc.gov/nchs/data/hus/hus05.pdf#029. The highway is more hostile to the very young, the very old and to impaired (drinking, drugs, disease) drivers http://www.cdc.gov/ncipc/duip/spotlite/teendrivers.htm http://www.cdc.gov/ncipc/factsheets/older.htm, http://www.cdc.gov/ncipc/duip/spotlite/3d.htm. These same risk factors make even our relatively safe home environment risky.

Falls just walking, on stairs, out windows or on ladders occur more with toddlers, the elderly and the impaired. Similarly swimming, boating, working, sports, hobbies, and other activities are all more dangerous for those groups. Intentional injuries may be controlled with improved technology, education on use of the technology and limiting access of high-risk groups to the technology. PHIT may be used to evaluate the safety of the technology with real time injury reporting, it may continually evaluate the users for their competence and capability in the technology before starting and with the use of web linked technology, it may adjust or limit the technology for high risk groups in real-time by disabling the technology or limiting maximum speeds or length or place of operation.

Intraspecies intentional injuries are due to competition for productive limited resources, territory and/or mates. There were 17,638 homicides in 2002.

http://www.cdc.gov/nchs/fastats/homicide.htm. 11,829 or 67% involved firearms. In 2003 for 10 to 24 year old people there were 5,570 homicides with 82% killed with firearms and 86% were males http://www.cdc.gov/ncipc/factsheets/yvfacts.htm. It is the leading cause of death for African American males in the 10 to 24 year old age group. In 2002 suicides caused 31,655 of the intraspecies violent deaths with 17,108 from firearms, 6,462 from suffocation and 5,489 from poisoning

http://www.cdc.gov/nchs/fastats/suicide.htm. Suicides usually occur when an environment with little available or enjoyable resources stresses someone with a genetic tendency to be depressed, cautious or anxious

http://www.ncbi.nlm.nih.gov/entrez/dispomim. cgi?id=608516. People without this tendency may overcome adversity with enhanced life skills if they survive the adverse environment. Adversity is in the eye of the beholder. We have a large amount of depression in the United States despite our affluence due to our high expectations. If more people had a global perspective and were able to avoid the unending commercial influence to consume foods and status symbols, we might be less depressed. Physical activity is also an antidote to depression. Our culture generally looks down on it with adverse consequences for our mental and physical health http://www.ncbi.nlm.nih.gov/entrez/query. fcgi?cmd=Retrieve&db=pubmed&dopt=Abstract&list_ uids=16534088&query_hl=7&itool=pubmed_docsum. This is the kids' version of the importance of exercise: http://kidshealth. org/kid/stay_healthy/fit/work_it_out.html.   Preventing homicides and suicides requires mental and social health interventions. Often teens with violent tendencies living in high risk areas may be spotted for special intervention http:// www.nlm.nih.gov/medlineplus/teenviolence.html#statistics.

http://www.ncbi.nlm.nih.gov/entrez/query. fcgi?cmd=Retrieve&db=pubmed&dopt=Abstract&list_ uids=14559956&query_hl=12&itool=pubmed_docsum   . Linking school, mental health, health, child abuse, and justice system information as much as allowed by law or by permission of the child and their custodian with the PHIT would help. TV watching tends to be associated with more violent ideas and aggressive behavior http://kidshealth.org/parent/positive/ family/tv_affects_child.html. Violent video games also increased aggressive behavior in youths http://www.ncbi.nlm.nih.gov/entrez/query. fcgi?cmd=Retrieve&db=pubmed&dopt=Abstract&list_ uids=16533123&query_hl=4&itool=pubmed_docsum.   TV shows, commercial advertisements, video games, movies, radio, drama, novels and graphic arts often use violence and sex to get our immediate interest. News programs often give notoriety to perpetrators of violence thereby indirectly rewarding it. Terrorist groups get publicity that may be used for recruiting future members. We do need to deal with these issues but when we just get bombarded with cheap distractions promoting some of our worst behaviors we likely suffer degradation of the quality of our lives and culture. Preventing homicides and suicides in an efficient manner would help conserve our human resources. Limiting gun access might delay deaths until therapy or social change might take place but would fail to eliminate the underlying problems that may manifest themselves in some other tool or means of destruction.

Some injuries are due to the combination of a hazardous environment and competition for resources. Teenagers may race cars to impress girls or to gain territory for their gang. Gun use by itself has some risks such as when hunting but is especially bad when used for fighting. Bullets may hit innocent bystanders with "friendly" fire. Cars, boats or other vehicles may be used as a form of territory that is mobile. Within the territory the operator may become too secure and get distracted from technical operations by sleeping, eating or interacting with others on the phone or in the car. Cars and other vehicles may be used as a weapon against rivals or as a way to commit suicide. We now have a disease syndemic http://www.cdc.gov/syndemics/index.htm of dangerous technology, rampant territory acquisition or commercialism, high-energy use in foods and transportation, and diminishing resources. Hopefully we may convert that to a health syndemic with safe technology, sharing to help the species, whole plant derived foods, transportation by muscle power when possible, and diminished pressure on limited resources.

Injuries are a major cause of death that needs to be addressed on a continuing basis as we change our way of living, our technology and our rivalries. Technologic fixes will help with unintentional injuries but social and mental health interventions will be needed to address the causes of intentional injuries.

CHAPTER 9
Mental Health: Dealing With Our Subconscious and Social Heritage

Our genetic heritage from our early vertebrate ancestors predisposes us to create and guard our territories and to mate. Our primate ancestors developed small social groups with hierarchies. Modern governments and cultures have superimposed complex social, technical and legal constraints on our daily lives. That only 49,000 out of 300 million people in the United States of America (USA) die intentionally each year, only 15% of elementary school children suffer from anxiety, only 3% of the population suffers from major psychological distress at any time is a major accomplishment of human adaptation of our old genetic tendencies, our old religions, our changing cultures and governments to a very new way of living. More simply put: mental illness is inevitable in these times since parents have to be a bit irrational to have kids. Parents have to be a bit emotional to want to put up with the care and feeding of dependents for a decade and then their financing until they become self-sufficient that might be another 21 years http://www.extension.umn.edu/distribution/businessmanagement/DF5899.html

http://www.cnpp.usda.gov/ExpendituresonChildrenbyFamilies.htm John Humphrey Noyes of the Oneida Community, Malthus, and the Shakers had also considered this extensively: http://libwww.syr.edu/digital/collections/m/MaleContinence-15k/. An emotional and religious view in favor of child rearing is presented here: http://www.lordoflifepc.org/CostofChildren. htm. Extreme mental illness with psychosis or depression that detaches the patient from reality or relating to people and often requires hospitalization, which occurs in about 1 in 200 people each year, is a detriment to having kids and caring for them. On the other hand pure rationality without any strong feelings may lead to a well performing member of society but is unlikely to lead to nesting and mating behavior when the world is already well populated and children are dependent for so long a time and their care is so expensive. As noted above many genes are related to anxiety, depression and neurotic behavior. This may be seen by searching OMIM (Online Mendelian Inheritance in Man) part of the National Library of Medicine Internet resources at http://www.ncbi.nlm.nih.gov/ entrez/query.fcgi?db=OMIM&itool=toolbar.

These traits probably all add to the strength of our territoriality proclivity that further enhances our chance to gain resources for mating and breeding and helps us respond to our mating urges. As may be seen by searches on these traits they are largely polygenetic with some expression with even one gene present. When we have one gene for anxiety, depression or neurotic behavior (the heterozygous condition) we may show some tendency for these behaviors when we are stressed or in a low resource situation. When we have 2 genes for any of these behaviors (the homozygous condition) we tend to get extreme in the behavior with even small amounts of stress. Dr E Creagan and E Sternberg write and talk about stress http://www.sciencefriday.com/program/archives/200711302 . At present and at least for the near foreseeable future we are unable to modify our own genes so the best we can do is to try to reduce our stress by changing our environment, lifestyle, and/or the way we think about what is happening to us.

Freud relegated to the subconscious id the defensive dark territorial forces and the light humanistic passionate forces. The ego keeps these subconscious forces from leading to self-destruction. The superego tries to make these forces socially useful by using morals and ethics http://en.wikipedia.org/wiki/Id%2C_ego%2C_and_super-ego .

These concepts are rooted in the 19th Century concepts of administration with bureaucracies being required to collect and disseminate or hide information to advance the state or corporation. Freud projects these external concepts to our brain's internal workings. Practically we balance these daily in work and play with a complex interplay between conscious and subconscious depending on the importance and complexity of the decisions. Now that technology allows we may take the connectedness and real-time functions of the brain that are adaptive and apply them to solve our problems by networking socially and/or electronically in real and virtual worlds.

Elliot Aronson notes how group or territorial feelings are so strong that they distort the way we interpret facts. This he calls cognitive dissonance http://www.npr.org/templates/story/story.php?storyId=12125926 . Without emotional involvement we may be more objective but we may then lack motivation. With emotions we may need special tools to be sure we are accurately observing the world and what it tells us about how we should live. For complex problems double blind randomized control trials are best when possible. Naturalized experiments may motivate them. http://www.pbs.org/wgbh/pages/frontline/shows/altmed/snake/research.html

The cautious, defensive, territorial and anxious child may be recognized easily. This child at 1 to 3 years of age hides under the chair or in the corner during doctor visits; usually avoids talking to strangers and hides from them; has a hard time getting to sleep without company; and clings to parents when sick or in a strange situation. In the school years the cautious child often cries at the beginning of the school year, avoids unusual activities, often complains of illness or bellyaches, and often misses school. When challenged, this child may regress and become defensive. In the teen and adult years the cautious child will have more risk of getting anxiety and depression. Some evidence exists that our territories are mapped into brain as written about by the Blakeslee's http://www.sciencefriday. com/program/archives/200712214 .

The brave, compassionate, outgoing, and adventurous child is quite a contrast. This child at 1 to 3 years old will greet and talk to health care providers; observes and talks to strangers; sleeps easily anywhere; and explores new environments eagerly. In school the brave child often finds new teachers and classes interesting, is rarely sick, and lacks complaints. When challenged, this child will try to rise to meet the new demands and will accept defeat graciously. In the teen and adult years the brave child will have more risk of injury and infectious disease from exploring new technology and environments.

By openly addressing our conscious and subconscious needs we may help reduce the energy sapping conflicts within ourselves. As noted above opening up our subconscious may unearth forces that we would usually like to avoid but dealing with them before they get in the way of our day to day social roles in society is helpful. We should recognize our primitive animal drives and appreciate how they helped our species and the biosphere get so far. We should avoid getting distracted by them or letting them lead us into unhealthy behavior. Often the arts help us deal with recognizing and expressing these feelings. Children who took drama lessons improved their social skills http://www.ncbi.nlm.nih.gov/entrez/query.fcgi?cmd=Retrieve&db=pubmed&dopt=Abstract&list_uids=15270994&query_hl=7&itool=pubmed_docsum. Music lessons in the same study improved the full scale IQ that helps us to be adaptive. Age and developmentally appropriate books, stories, art appreciation, plays, radio, music, TV and movies may also be helpful. Religion helps through giving us time proven stories to help us understand and deal with life. All cultures believe in a God or Gods. I am unable to prove the existence of any God but I may prove to you that sustainable human cultures tend to believe in at least one. It likely relates to the social hierarchies in our primate groups. We tend to look to a leader and given our cynicism and intelligence we quickly realize that our self and other humans are inadequate to the task. Our God or Gods serve as the ultimate leader or leading group who will guide our religion and culture to success in survival. Modern religions recognize that God or Gods speak to us through history with our failures such as 9/11 and HIV, showing us paths to avoid; and our successes, such as micro loans and truthful education to stimulate the economies of the developing and developed world, show us the ways to seek. With world travel, commerce and communication we will need to create a contemporary world religion that encompasses all the good of the world and helps synthesize a new believable story of how we relate to each other and our Gods or Gods. Stories about species development, adaptation and survival would be nice but may fail to meet our primal needs for the story to involve some human like leader figure or a family of characters. Now culture often just defaults to commercial interests dominating our relationships and that has failed to be adequate in the past and will likely be inadequate in its pure form for long-term goals and relations. Joseph Campbell has written extensively about creating myths and religions http://www.jcf.org/index2.php. The tower of Babel and the World Trade Center as vertical structures or any vertical human hierarchy such as a multinational corporation or a centrally controlled super power may fail to adapt to all the unique religious, cultural and environmental conditions around the world http://www.commongood.info/. Vertical structures are also vulnerable to terrorism or natural disasters due to dependence on each link in the structure remaining intact. Horizontal infrastructure that connects interactively with information sharing to help direct resources to where they are most needed and find products where they are best produced would likely be most helpful. Horizontal infrastructures may fill in from all sides whenever one link is destroyed or inoperable. The Internet as a horizontal structure constantly adjusts to find the fastest route for information packets almost instantaneously. Renewable decentralized power sources called micro power with horizontal distribution would add stability to our society http://www. amazon.com/gp/product/0374236755/sr=1-2/qid=1154873257/ ref=pd_bbs_2/104-7004443-3374348?ie=UTF8&s=books and

http://www.vijaytothepeople.com/. A diet with locally grown whole plant derived foods would be secure in most situations. Communications must respect the feelings of all involved and yet be open enough to be helpful to all to adapt to a changing environment. The Internet when used by thoughtful culturally sensitive people is very helpful but as with any technology it may also be misused for censorship and unfeeling and uninformed central control. As the USA Constitution states vertical or central federal powers should be limited for self-defense from other vertical powers and other essential national government concerns such as interstate and international commerce. The Constitution allows for states, religions and groups of the people to adapt and organize in diverse ways as they choose to best suit the needs and beliefs of their members.

To start on the path to optimal mental health we must evaluate our basic needs to survive and develop species promoting well functioning adult humans. Optimal mental health promotes species survival through helping individual adapt to their best role in this endeavor. Children should be taught practical social and self-care skills. As they mature their natural talents should be guided to full development in some useful social role. Religion or spiritual development formal or informal may provide useful stories to give meaning to the lives of children and adults. Current secular divorces just put monetary values on the family that fail to recognize spiritual commitments. Forced marriages or marriages that are undissolvable have lead to much violence in the past and should also be avoided. We should realize that we in the USA are at present blessed with huge amounts of wealth and resources compared with the rest of the world's population. We should us these resources to learn more of our world and ourselves. This will help guide us to plan for the future of our species. Our communications, transportation and energy infrastructure is amazing though vulnerable. We need to add to our decentralized capabilities to deal with problems when central control or power is inaccessible. We should develop efficient transportation that may be hydrogen or human powered or powered by some other renewable resource. Energy production from decentralized stores of hydrogen or other renewable efficient source should at least be available for emergencies and used whenever it is more efficient. Human sources of energy will also help encourage us to exercise for physical and mental health. Food stores and fast food are centralized too often. Many inner city neighborhoods lack any ready source of vegetables and fruits. Insecurity about food with much of our supplies coming from distant parts of the country or unknown or unseen nearby places may add to our tendency to anxiety and to overeat. Psychological studies have shown that watching food on Television (TV) tends to make us hungrier and to eat more. Smelling food and farms tends to make us eat less. People who watch more TV tend to be more overweight

http://www.nlm.nih.gov/medlineplus/ency/article/001999.htm.

This may give body image and self-esteem problems. Fast foods promote maximum calorie consumption with minimum vegetable use, that is fine for the under weight vegetable eaters but 30% of us now are overweight and many of use eat too few vegetables. Nutrition and cooking are poorly taught at home and just given token attention at most schools. Kids who sit down to dinner with their family usually eat better and do better with mental tasks but family meals are increasingly rare

http://www.mayoclinic.com/health/healthy-diet/NU00190

http://www.hsph.harvard.edu/nutritionsource/pyramids.html.

Once the family has prepared the child physically and mentally for formal education the schools should help the child develop to his or her potential. Before the 1800's formal schooling was optional with most children educated simply at home or church. Privileged youth were taught reading, writing, and arithmetic, with only the very privileged going on to advanced work in college and the learned professions. Compulsory education that developed by the 1900's has allowed youth to benefit from education with better skills and mental tools for dealing with our complex world but it has also created anxiety and stress for some youth that lacks the interest or capability to learn in school. About 50% of high school students have some neurological learning deficit but only 10% have any problems. The 40% with a neurological learning deficit and without manifest problems have learned to compensate through their own experience. At least 3% of youth have failed to make it to the high school level due to extreme intelligence problems. Melvin Levine, MD has written and talked about these problems extensively: http://www.retctrpress.com/Authors/levine.php. There are of course many others in school who lack motivation or a cultural understanding. In the past these youth learned through apprenticeship or work. Schools now provide vocational training but often are disconnected from employers and workforce realities. Paul Goodman in the 1960's noted the stress caused by the standard education system that fails to adapt to individual needs:

http://dwardmac.pitzer.edu/Anarchist_Archives/bright/goodman/goodman-bio.html. Since then we have had legislation mandating Individual Education Plans (IEP's) for students with special needs but schools still orient largely to the average student, with still much anxiety and depression caused in students that are different. School bureaucracies with unions and tenure policies often make it hard for schools to adapt http://www.empirepage.com/guesteds/guesteds328.html. Many great figures have had atypical educational patterns. Andrew Carnegie learned through work and self-study. He went on to create the USA steel industry and later supported education through philanthropy http://en.wikipedia.org/wiki/Andrew_Carnegie.

Thomas Edison was a failure in school but was taught by his mother who was trained as a teacher http://en.wikipedia.org/wiki/Thomas_Edison. Sean Connery dropped out of school as a teenager and learned acting through work and practice http://www.seanconnery.com/biography/. These people had some protection from anxiety through their beliefs and/or genes. When adversity occurred they persevered, as the heroes of Joseph Campbell, rather than succumbing to depression or fear or defense of a limited territory http://www.pbs.org/moyers/faithandreason/perspectives1.html .

Children and adults need to see something more to life than their immediate gratification to avoid self-destruction through over indulgence or hurting others through violent or psychological abuse (as in the 12 Step Program used by AA and others http://en.wikipedia.org/wiki/12_step). Religious confirmation, outward bound, or challenging and meaningful work experiences often gives youth a spiritual rite of passage that makes them feel part of the adult community http://en.wikipedia.org/wiki/Rite_of_passage . Frank Schaeffer in AWOL argues for 2 to 3 years of community or military service for all youths to help the USA and help give a sense of belonging and purpose to the youths http://www.frankschaeffer.net/awol.html. Without these programs many youth use gang or fraternity hazing to get their rite of passage. Often simple commercial secularism fails to suffice.

For others with anxiety or depression and less skill sets; improving their economic or community environment may help their behavior. In a rural poverty area of the South East USA a casino operated by American Indians opened up in the middle of a study doing regular psychiatric health assessments from

1993 to 2000. Youths in families benefiting from improved income or jobs still had symptoms of anxiety and depression but had less conduct and oppositional defiant symptoms. Their genetic tendencies for anxiety and depression persisted while their behavior moderated perhaps due to less desperation http://www.ncbi.nlm.nih.gov/entrez/query.fcgi?cmd=Retrieve&db=pubmed&dopt=Abstract&list_uids=14559956&query_hl=3&itool=pubmed_docsum. Of course this is a relative economic problem with even the poor in the USA having more than most other people in the world but we in the USA expect more. Traditional cultures may also keep their values better with people more convinced of the meaning of their life. Other cultures are freer of commercial distractions and the fostering of our attention on costly things that work against our own good and the good of our community such as greed, gluttony and our immediate self-gratification. Most other cultures have lower rates of mental illness than we do in the USA: 26% of USA residents have had a mental disorder in the past year versus only 5% of the residents of Nigeria, 8% of Italians, 12% of Mexicans, 15% of Netherlanders, and 18% of French, http://www.msnbc.msn.com/id/5111202 and JAMA: http://www.ncbi.nlm.nih.gov/entrez/query.fcgi?cmd=Retrieve&db=pubmed&dopt=Abstract&list_uids=15173149&query_hl=8&itool=pubmed_docsum. With TV, radio and newspapers we are constantly given news to be anxious about while we worry about how many consumer products we lack. Many brave immigrants initially settled the USA. Our bias to change and our striving for better things and ways of living may also create more stress and anxiety.

Do we worry too much or too little? Only the future will tell. Our biologic and social diversity creates people with different outlooks and attitudes. The ones that worry the right amount about the right problems will survive the best. For our species it is good to have 25% of people that are very cautious, 50% that are fairly cautious and 25% that are brave with much lack of genetic cautiousness. The brave individuals will explore and experiment but often these adventures may end up in disaster so the cautious core will survive and carry on our species. If the brave are successful they will expand our species into new environments and bring the species new resources that have never before been used such as new foods or other energy supplies. The fairly cautious group will change over 1 to 4 years so they might avoid injury if the disastrous consequences of a change are delayed such as by slow poisoning in the new food or the new technology; or from unusual but dire consequences of a new environment such as earthquakes, fires, or plagues. The very cautious may be holding onto their old ways for even a generation so they would still survive. This may explain the high degree of anxiety and depression amongst Native American Indians. Many of the brave ones actively fought Western Europeans and were destroyed leaving a higher percentage of the very cautious amongst the survivors. After our wars we suffer depression from the loss of loved ones but also the population loses many resilient brave ones. One reaction to guilt and Post Traumatic Stress Disorder (PTSD) is alcoholism that may increase after wars http://www.ncptsd. va.gov/ncmain/ncdocs/fact_shts/fs_alcohol.html?opm=1&rr= rr95&srt=d&echorr=true. These differences in cautiousness seem to involve most vertebrates, and have benefited our large biologic group and the biosphere through increased adaptability with fail-safe stability.

Individuals with strong genetic tendencies to be cautious or brave will be more susceptible to mental illness when stressed.

The very cautious when put in an adverse environment may become paranoid and if obsessed with their fears may become separated from reality. Less extreme problems would be anxiety and depression. When controlled the cautious tendency may help conserve traditional attributes that are healthy and adaptive but may be ignored by the current culture. The extremely brave when stressed may become megalomaniacs or over egotistical if they survive. When more controlled they may be anti-social or misbehave more often while being creative and taking risks. When well controlled they may be our well-socialized soldiers and explorers taking risks for society and culture. Even with a well functioning brain we may have problems achieving a balance of our individual view of the world and our given place in it. When an illness caused by an infection, by toxins or drugs inhibits the brain function we often will have more problems.

In the past and present we try to control drugs that may be toxic. Drugs toxic in large amounts or when addiction occurs may be helpful in small amounts by decreasing anxiety or by stimulating attention. In Russia in 1914 the Czar with the backing of the church prohibited alcohol use to promote better discipline and morality in Russian men and army in World War I. It was a big change that in part brought on the Communist Revolution with alcohol. Alcohol in moderate amounts does decrease shame http://www.tomkins.org/home/ and alcohol fermented drinks often contain antibiotics to help fight germs. Before 1920 there now no known antibiotics. Such a sudden cultural change, however well meaning, was hard for Russia and the USA to take. In the USA the right of women to vote was resisted in part due to the strong Women's Christian Temperance Union (WCTU). Politicians knew that if women were given the right to vote they would soon bring on prohibition. This would help decrease some of the abuse of women and children but would remove the main financial support of the Federal Government. Up to 1920 the USA Federal Government's main revenue was from taxes on alcoholic beverages. With prohibition income taxes had to be drastically increased. With prohibition crime to support the ingrained drinking habit and disease from tainted or toxic unregulated alcohol products increased. Fortunately our Constitution allows change so our government survived by just repealing the Constitutional Amendment. Both countries showed that in the early 1900's some brave social engineers and intellectuals thought that we could simply try to change human behavior by law without some dire consequences. For the past 30 years we try to control cocaine and heroin only to benefit our favorite war lords who fought the Soviet Union in Afghanistan or the communists in Central America http://ciadrugs.homestead. com/files/index.html , http://www.ciadrugs.com/ . Without these sanctioned drug sales we may have been unable to afford to fight Soviets and other communists. We do support the illusion that controlling drugs from communists or terrorists is good for our country but lose it when we benefit from drug sales by war loads that are fighting terrorists or religious extremists hostile to the USA. We need to face the fact that often the ends do not justify the means. The means in this case corrupts and destroys the society and citizens of the USA, though in the short run meeting some foreign policy objectives. Perhaps drugs like alcohol are best used when highly regulated and taxed to prevent them from benefiting illegal or terrorists groups and harming innocents with the monitoring of the health and the delivery of care done by PHIT (Public Health Information Technology). Information systems with Bioidentifiers, identity cards, and passwords may help intelligently regulate all addictive habits and substances. To best control alcohol, drug, food, gambling, and sex misuse, we must develop a strong culture and religion encouraging human development and cooperation that will help alleviate anxiety and depression and direct human exploration in positive directions.

We have used rituals and drugs to deal with mental illness from the beginning of our species. Primates and birds seek social ritual comfort in stress http://www.sciencefriday.com/newsbriefs/read/141. In ancient Egypt physicians would use incantations to help people feel better. This may have helped anxious people to relax and allow for natural healing. Magic wands with hieroglyphs representing the goddess Taweret, part hippopotamus, were used to draw circles of protection around infant cribs. This created a magical protective territory http://www.metmuseum.org/special/Art_Medicine_Egypt/view_1.asp?item=4 . Fermented alcoholic drinks for adults often contained antibiotics and helped some to relieve their shame and anxiety temporarily. Mentally ill within small groups were recognized as different and would fill some limited special social roles. If they were dangerous they were expelled to the wilderness to protect the social group. In the past few hundred years for people harmful to themselves or others we have tried special institutions or hospitals to remove the mentally ill from cities with some success. Now we often use medications to decrease the harm that the mentally ill might do to themselves or others while remaining in the community. Even some bears know to eat special plants if they are sick. Deer will go to saltlicks to get minerals. Some medications help with improving concentration and attitude. All have some side effects. They usually are less harmful than alcoholic intoxication, narcotics, stimulants or smoking. Of course we still use counseling and social supports to guide the anxious and misbehaving to acceptable norms. In the early 1900's we emphasized problems derived from sexual inhibitions and obsessions as discussed by Sigmund Freud but in the mid 1950's the Tompkins Institute corrected psychological theory by noting many other things that humans find interesting and the importance of subconscious social interactions starting even in infancy http://www.behavior.net/column/nathanson/bio.html. Pets have helped with our security in the past. Dogs guard and control livestock and act as organic burglar alarms. Dalmatian dogs tend to bite and bark and get along well with horses so were used to guard the horses of fire companies in the 1800's. Even when the horses left fireman still continued to keep them, as watchdogs for facilities were people were often coming and going on rapid notice. Cats do well in guarding grain stores, food and kitchens from rodents. We may continue to enjoy our warm furry protective systems better than electronic protective systems and chemical exterminators. Pets may give some relief from anxiety by their attentiveness to our needs and their ancient relations with humans. We still have much to learn in dealing with individual mental health problems and they best treatment. PHIT with continuous evaluation of our treatments and their results is needed.

Our culture has further suffered and benefited from cautiousness and braveness. In the early 1900's city planners were predicting a catastrophe in the 1920's when the amount of horse manure that cities would produce would exceed the capacity of the cities to remove it. Of course the automobile and trucks solved that one but came up with new forms of pollutions and injuries. In the mid 1970's Dr. David Sencer was the head of the CDC http://www.cdc.gov/about/pastdirectors6. htm and was concerned that swine flu or swine influenza would infect the population of the USA causing a pandemic http://www.cdc.gov/ncidod/EID/vol8no8/01-0474.htm. There were only a few human cases but he knew then as we know now that an influenza outbreak may become a severe pandemic causing the permanent loss of up to 1% of healthy productive adults and short term severe illness in 30% of the population http://www.cdc.gov/flu/pandemic/keyfacts.htm. So he decided to create a vaccine for swine flu and offer it to all in the USA. I'm brave so I got mine in 1976. About one in 100,000 people got Guillain Barre Syndrome after getting the vaccine and swine flu failed to be a problem. After leaving the CDC in 1977 Dr. David Sencer then became the director of the NY City Department of Health. He was present in the early 1980's when young men with frequent drug use and frequent sexual contacts started getting immune deficiency problems. Perhaps his adverse experience with reacting to swine flu colored his response these first AIDS (Acquired Immunodeficiency Syndrome) cases. He may have wanted to avoid over reacting to a disease that may have also failed to spread like swine flu. The NYC gay community was also against an aggressive and possibly punitive disease control measures so any efforts to control AIDS in its earliest stages would have required great and extremely tactful political efforts. Unfortunately diseases are often unique and unpredictable. Of course AIDS went on to kill millions and swine flu so far remains quiescent. Since the 1940's we have worried about nuclear weapons with much efforts coming from the cautious in resisting their acceptance as standard weapons and the brave in finding new ways to control them with civil disobedience and political action. So far we have had success.

In the future we will need to deal with challenging issues such as fluoride, global warming, energy use, terrorism and centralization with the right mixture of caution and experimentation. Fluoride use in public water supplies has helped decrease tooth decay that causes pain and suffering, but there is a risk of perhaps an extra 1 case in 100,000 boys of osteosarcoma or bone cancer from the current use of fluoride http://www.cdc.gov/oralhealth/waterfluoridation/index.htm. Osteosarcoma may be fatal and at least debilitating for 1 to 2 years http://www.fluorideaction.org/. Should we increase the chance that a very small number of children would get bone cancer in order to protect a large number of children and adults from dental disease? Should we just invest more in getting children and adults to take better care of their teeth and eat better foods even though this would cost 10 to 100 times more than just using fluoride? For the cautious the answer is simply to stop any interventions that might be harmful since the anxiety is too great to be worth it. For the brave the answer is to try what helps the most people since they rarely worry. For 50% with some anxiety the logic is uncertain. For most for us we need more information with continuous analysis of how we use fluoride and what kind of results we get. Using PHIT (Public Health Information Technology) will help us make some sense out of this problem.

Similar conundrums involving global warming, nuclear energy, the control of terrorism and the decentralization of resources challenge us. If we continue to ignore these issues or address them inadequately mental stress will continue to increase. Our current commercial culture concentrates on the ephemeral with little help to those that need direction and meaning in their life to ward off anxiety, anger and depression.

In the USA and in many areas of the world young adults with average skills and education find it difficult to earn a living, support a small family and enjoy life http://www.nytimes. com/2006/06/25/business/yourmoney/25view.html?ex=115207 2000&en=1a054d6d101ef5a3&ei=5070&emc=eta1, while the richest 1% of the population gets much richer and we worry about abolishing a tax for the richest 0.5% http://www.npr. org/templates/story/story.php?storyId=4725777. With global warming we wonder if we should continue to enjoy so far relatively cheap fossil fuel or change over sooner to renewable energy resources that fail to produce much carbon dioxide. Some scenarios may be disastrous as in bringing on catastrophic tides, weather, and perhaps a new ice age. It costs us in terms of real and intellectual resources to change our infrastructure more quickly and perhaps with little benefit. Nuclear energy may give us short-term cheaper energy but in the long run in the unknown future will likely cost us more in safety and health or in confining radioactivity. Controlling terrorism will require greater control of communications: electronic, digital, and mail; and the movement of people and potential weapons. We must weigh the cost of the loss of some privacy and freedom against the cost of destruction by committed intelligent groups and individuals that are opposed to our society and other world societies. How much should we decentralize to avoid the severe consequences of natural and man-made disasters? Is the loss of central control and efficiencies of scale worth the increased security and ease of communications when power and intellect are dispersed? To deal with these issues and many others we need the best and most current information available with continuing reevaluations done as we choose different interventions in order to best adapt our species to our biosphere. Using PHIT with population and environmental analysis will help us adapt. Now when people and governments seemingly ignore these problems it increases the anxiety levels and despair of any sensitive souls. Too much information may also be incapacitating to those that get upset easily. With Internet information systems not only should we be able to choose the security of the computer but also we should be able to choose information at the scare levels that we find the most comfortable. When threats become more real and less theoretical we must inform even the most anxious.

Complicating our medical, social, religious, environmental and energy problems is the ancient vertebrate phenomena of territories. To build a therapeutic society that comforts and supports our anxious and helps our distracted to concentrate on important goals we need to understand our basic vertebrate tendencies. Dogs mostly urinate for marking purposes at significant landmarks. Cats like rubbing their chin on things or people that they would to possess. Birds mostly use songs and displays to mark their space to control the resources for nesting and breeding http://www.animalbehavioronline.com/9.html and http://www.stanford.edu/group/stanfordbirds/text/essays/Territoriality.html. Human individuals have different kinds of territories. Sometimes it is concrete like the man or woman whose home is his or her castle or child whose room is his or her castle. For these people moving or having relatives or worse strangers moving in with them is very threatening. Sometimes territory may be abstract such in stored treasure or money that gives some a feeling of security, or even more abstract as a skill or intellectual area of expertise. In homes changes in cooking or recycling may be threatening to older family members especially the cautious. At work bureaucrats or technicians in organizations guard their skill areas from encroachments and keep special information to themselves. Any changes may produce much more stress than the simple problem of learning new ways of doing things. Sharing information and resources to help people and the organization adapt, is threatening many people. We must balance a tendency to care for our family, and group; against a tendency to gain and protect territory. In extreme either tendency may be bad with narcissism and ethnocentricism; or greed and hoarding. The natural experiment that increased incomes to a poor population may have helped reduce acting out and behavioral problems by expanding the virtual territory of the poor families. Primitive territorial phenomena such as marking prized areas with disgusting scents may be seen in toddlers, and in uncontrolled youths and adults. More commonly verbal allusions to scenting substances and mating practices are used to evoke the emotional strength of the defense or the defining of a territory. In the Wild West style of Internet of today we may have virtual territory at our Web Page or in our e-mail with virus and worm creators continually trying to invade our territory and spam creators trying to use our territory to their gain. In the future a secure Internet may help protect medical, economic, public safety and defense information while an insecure Internet may exist separately as a playground for intellectual games and for those anxious about their privacy as long as they fail to threaten other real people. Celebrity or notoriety may be seen as an expansion of virtual territory in the media of story, newspaper, radio, TV, Internet, or movies. Good behaviors should be noted and people should be warned of bad behavior, but we must be careful that falsehoods are detected and that bad individuals fail to benefit from publicity.

Societies around the world often exclude non-members from or foreigners from resources and privileges. In medical care we try to be culturally sensitive to help the ill. In society we should value appropriately all the contributors to help them feel wanted and secure. In the USA being started by immigrants and refugees and having abundant untapped resources we have been the most open and accepting society but we still have limits. In the early 1900's we limited immigrants and even excluded Asians. Now illegal aliens or immigrants make up about 10% of our work force. We on one hand would like to keep foreigners out of our territory but on the other hand we do not want to pay higher wages and benefits to workers so as to attract USA citizens or legal immigrants to the lowest level jobs. So far our poor lack of border and resident control allows us to claim we protect our territory to make the ultra territorial people feel better and allow aliens to be discriminated against yet allows business and labor to function to meet market demands. As we protect ourselves from terrorism with better identification of people and products, then we must give some legal status to so many people that help to run our country and who would like to help our country develop. Similarly illegal drugs and merchandise that may serve some useful role in society should be taxed and regulated to benefit those who might need them and to restrict them from those who might be harmed. With bioidentification, bar codes and RFID (Radio Frequency Identification Devices) integrated into PHIT we should easily be able to administer guest worker, pre-citizens or legal immigrant worker programs while identifying criminal or terrorist persons or merchandise such as drugs or weapons of domestic or foreign origin that should be confined and/or controlled. Many of our confined domestic and alien population suffers from adaptation, mental health and/or drug problems that might be better handled and for less cost through well controlled therapeutic interventions closely monitored by

PHIT with GPS (global positioning systems) in cell phones that would allow for automated supervision of individuals with significant behavioral problems.

The religions of Christianity, Muslimism, and Buddhism are abstract and only indirectly attached to a geographic region. They have just originated in the past two thousand years with elements of older religions synthesized into them. They tend to promote and reward the universal virtues of a spiritual life and helping our fellow humans. Karen Armstrong notes the new emphasis on compassion (an ancient vertebrate and mammalian trait http://www.npr.org/templates/story/story.php?storyId=5534300) and empathy coming out of the religions in the Axial Age 2500 years ago http://www.npr.org/templates/story/story.php?storyId=5307044 . At that time the efficiency of the newly developed iron weapons threatened to destroy society if left unchecked by nonviolent action http://en.wikipedia.org/wiki/Axial_Age. Despite this, these and other religions have been constrained by nationalism or extremist sects and commandeered to fit the needs of territorialism. In the 1600's to the 1800's Roman Catholic and Protestant Christians often fought to the death, just as Muslim Shiites and Sunnis fight today. Karen Armstrong describes this as the preference for people for righteousness over compassion. Righteousness is intellectual territorialism that is harmful in science; culture, government and religion when it keeps us from adapting though in moderation it may be helpful in identifying the best quality information. In World Wars I and II American, English and German Christians were told God was on their side despite their worshipping the same God as their opponents worshipped. Karen Armstrong sees fundamentalism as starting in the USA as a social reaction against the rapidly changing world of the

Industrial and Scientific Revolution. Fundamentalists protect the territory of old ideas and practices against new science, technology and ways of life that bring with them the stress and anxiety of change. The forces of territory may be very strong. Some people such as Professor Daniel Dennett advocate teaching more about the history and traditions of religion in order to prevent people from using religion as an excuse for war http://www.aarp.org/fun/radio/pt_radio/faith_and_fact.html, http://en.wikipedia.org/wiki/Daniel_Dennett. Jonathan Miller further expounds on the problems of religion in his 3 part TV series "A Brief History of Disbelief" http://www.pbs.org/moyers/journal/blog/2007/05/a_brief_history_of_disbelief.html.

If only logic were enough this would suffice but in any case it may help for many, and inspire others to identify with the earth as a single territory.

Once we achieve that viewpoint we may still have a problem. Humans often see the earth as one territory to exploit for the short-term gains of our species. When we are species centric we may fail to note that we still have much interdependence with other species in the biosphere. If too much of the rain forest is destroyed we may have more carbon dioxide and less oxygen. If global warming upsets the Gulf Stream we may get colder in Northern Europe and North America and upset the circulation of nutrients from the ocean floor to the surface waters thereby decreasing fish populations. Humans are important but without the biosphere existing in a form that we may adapt to, we may fail to survive. We are often unable to predict what will happen but we should plan for the worst and hope for the best. Our species may depend on that.

Giant coal and petrochemical corporations now mostly control energy sources. We have a model of centralized mass produced resources controlled by a few mega corporations. President George W. Bush's administration has chosen to emphasize doubts about global warming despite real concerns about it happening and its possible catastrophic effects http://www.climatecrisis.net/thescience/. In the 1970's our nuclear engineer President Jimmy Carter tried start us down the road to using renewable resources. Our economy suffered as would be expected and our citizens were unwilling to pay the price for decreased oil dependence. In his book, Power to the People, Vijay Vaitheeswaran describes how we may have done better and may yet do better to achieve energy independence http://www.amazon.com/gp/product/0374236755/sr=1-2/qid=1154205688/ref=pd_bbs_2/103-1733450-9433442?ie=UTF8&s=books. Now the Department of Defense has paid for a study by Amory Lovins to decrease our dependence on oil http://www.oilendgame.com/. Ethanol from corn may help us for emergencies if our foreign oil supplies are cut off but over the next 10 to 20 years it would waste about as much oil as it saves. This is a recent discussion from NPR http://www.sciencefriday.com/pages/2007/Oct/hour1_100407.html. Willows and switch grass only do slightly better. Colin Campbell notes that going to a whole food plant derived diet will make us much healthier and save on energy and other environmental resources http://www.thechinastudy.com/. With the use of drug and tax money President Reagan defeated Communism and the Soviet Union with the undesired side effect of continued oil addiction and promotion of extreme fundamentalist Muslim religious groups. These Muslim extremist freedom fighters helped us defeat the Soviet Union in Afghanistan then went on to attack our capitalist promotion of the Western hedonistic life style. Osama bin Laden and his Islamic Sunni fundamentalist Taliban allies were our allies in that conflict with the Soviet Union but were always resistant the Western tolerance of nudity, alcohol and non-traditional living of young adults outside of families and marriage. The fundamentalist Sunni religious supported by oil wealth from Saudi Arabia promote opposition and hatred in an environment full of biased information about the West and moderate Muslimism. They are creating their own regional and religious territory. Our response has been territorial with invasions of their geography and attempts to control the country and perhaps the oil of Iraq. We may do better by recognizing the universal commonalities of the conservative religious of the USA, Britain, and the Middle East http://pewglobal.org/americaagainsttheworld/. All emphasize the spiritual and long-term goals of humans and de-emphasize short-term economic gains. Unfortunately so far it has always been difficult except in the times of extreme crisis to get much political support in the USA for self-sacrifice now for future generations. The stress of 9/11 reinforced the old fashioned territoriality of the Neocons that resonated with our vertebrate past. To resist such temptations we truly need extensive and accurate international systems of information with a deep understanding of our adversaries. USA government's statements distorted even short-term obvious facts. Al Qaeda was said to be in Iraq before the USA invasion despite meager evidence for it and much against it http://www.pbs.org/wgbh/pages/frontline/darkside/view/. Our long term past support of Saddam Hussein in Iraq fighting Iran and Osama bin Laden in Afghanistan fighting the Soviets were conveniently forgotten. Our support of USA corporations to the detriment of the health and well being of foreign countries works against stable world security and peace though often profitable to us in the short run http://

www.johnperkins.org/. Education in foreign languages and cultures for our students with the exchange of students and educational support for students in foreign lands to learn about our history in an unbiased manner would likely help, but has decrease since 9/11 2001. Gene Sharp has documented many non-violent techniques to change governments and has helped guide the USA http://en.wikipedia.org/wiki/Gene_Sharp. These techniques would have less adverse side effects than war. The orthodox left has been upset with Professor Sharp for consulting with Defense Department of the USA. I believe this is because the left claims nonviolence as its intellectual territory and is threatened in its primitive vertebrate core when others invade without paying homage or dues to its non-establishment establishment http://www.voltairenet.org/article30032.html. Perhaps we should encourage a good means even when our intellectual opponents use it. If the left and the right both encourage changes supported by truth that most people accept, and will work for them for different theoretical reasons this would likely be an adaptive change for our species. Changes helping both people and commerce are possible. A Force More Powerful dramatizes non-violent action in a video game and a movie http://www.afmpgame.com/, http://www.aforcemorepowerful.org/. Counterinsurgency, the field manual from the United States Army, promotes non-violent techniques with armed force only as the last resort http://www.fas.org/irp/doddir/army/fm3-24fd.pdf. We should continually try to improve our information on foreign and domestic policies, intervene in the best way possible, and reevaluate to improve our future legitimate and socially acceptable interventions. Territorial functions that help to protect and distribute economic and intellectual resources must be balanced with compassion for those in need. PHIT or other accessible yet secure information systems may help on an international basis to distribute resources for all peoples and countries in a fair, compassionate and adaptive manner.

CHAPTER 10
Biohazards: Toxins, Excess Energy, and Germs

The environment affects us with every photon or particle of radiation, with every air movement, with each breath, with each swallow and with close body contacts. We have adapted so that most of these interactions are favorable to us. With changes in the environment due to ecosystem or biosphere changes or due to our movement out of our old environment and into a new environment we become exposed to possibly toxic new physical agents. For psychologically sensitive people, just being in a new environment creates anxiety and stress; even though it may prove beneficial when they lose their worries. Some changes may be natural and gradual so that we may adapt easily; or some may be catastrophic and sudden such as hurricanes or terrorist attacks. Some changes may be brought about by humans using new technology to extend our ability to move into new environments and use new resources or some may be brought by competing humans trying to eliminate rivals for scarce resources and territory.

We are continuously bathed by radiation. Some we see such as visible light and some at wavelengths that are too short to see such as x-ray or that are too long to see such as infrared, microwaves, radar, and radio waves. Photons or sunlight helps our skin to produce Vitamin D that gives us strong bones, healthy muscles, decreases allergies and helps our pancreas prevent diabetes, but too much sun may burn.

Where we evolved originally in Africa near the equator we had dark skin to prevent burns. As we moved away from the equator only those with light skin that could produce more Vitamin D survived well so our skin became lighter in those regions over hundreds of thousands of years. Now diminishing ozone layers in the atmosphere may increase irritation and cancer risk from sunlight. Radiation from x-rays, nuclear fuel, nuclear weapons, nuclear waste, or naturally occurring radon gas may all causes destruction of cells and over many years cancer. These forms of radiation are undetectable to our senses. Current diagnostic x-ray technology is much better than in the 1920's when it was first used. Then often patients and physicians would get overdosed with resulting skin burns or damage from simple x-rays to look at lungs, heart and bones. Radiologists in the early years had increased cancer rates. New machines and technology use less radiation to the patient to get better images with the help of more sensitive x-ray film and digital or electronic sensors and computer analysis. X-rays from the sun hit us all the time. The radiation we receive from the sun over a one-year period amounts to what we might get from 2 chest x-ray studies. The earth's electromagnetic field shields us from much radiation. In highflying airplanes on polar routes, we receive increased radiation and in space in an unshielded craft we might receive toxic amounts of radiation from the occasional sun spot activity or solar storms or coronal mass ejections (CME's) http://solar.physics.montana.edu/press/WashPost/Horizon/1961-031099-idx.html. Radon is radioactive gas that is present in many geologic formations including coal and shale. In small concentrations it has little radioactivity but if it builds up inside of mines or in basements or homes it may increase your risk of lung cancer. Special monitoring kits available from some health departments and some hardware

or home supply stores may be used to detect it http://www.
nyhealth.gov/nysdoh/radon/radonhom.htm. Microwaves or
radar ranges that have been heating our food since the 1950's
are safe with shielding. Microwaves in humans in low amounts
might produce mild warming but in large amounts would
cause heat damage or burning. Electromagnetic radiation
from electric blankets or high-powered electronic transmission
lines might be cause a slight risk of cancer but not much more
than the risk that most of us experience. Our main day-to-
day risk in this area is with sunburn depending on how light
colored our skin is. Light colored skin allows for more vitamin
D production that enabled survival of humans in areas of the
world away from the equator though it increases the risk of
sunburn and skin cancer. Our main catastrophic risk would be
from nuclear war, terrorism or faulty technology leading to the
release of large amounts of radiation. War and terrorism need
to be controlled with the development of world diplomacy and
religion. We need wide spread real time defense and security
systems that monitor radiation and connect with PHIT (Public
Health Information Technology) and identify persons that may
transport or work with radioactive substances all over the world.
We need to closely inventory and control radioactive materials
all over the world without threatening the ancient territorial
fears of developing nations and established world powers. This
will take a great deal of tact and restraint by the USA who as
the lone super power is perceived as very threatening by most
other nations and social groups throughout the world.

Controlling and monitoring nuclear power and its by
products to prevent melt downs and low grade environmental
degradation requires eternal vigilance (or at least for 10,000
years worth of monitoring). With nuclear power plant

accidents; such as at Chernobyl in the Ukraine and Three Mile Island in Pennsylvania, USA; and with some types of dirty bombs made from power plant waste radioactive iodine may be released. Taking large amounts of potassium iodine before getting exposed to the radioactive iodine will help protect the thyroid by blocking the uptake of the radioactive iodine by saturating the thyroid with non-radioactive iodine. This helps to prevent thyroid cancer. For other radioactive elements we lack any specific preventive measures besides avoid exposure and especially ingestion of the radioactive material. For more specifics see the CDC (Centers for Disease Control and Prevention) site http://www.bt.cdc.gov/radiation/.

Extremes in heat or cold are fatal. In the North of the USA we often say it is as cold as hell and in the South we often say it is as hot as hell. Either extreme will cause suffering. Larger humans have less surface area per volume so lose less heat in a cold environment. Generally people who have lived in colder areas for millennia tend to be larger and that likely has helped them survive the frigid weather. Babies and children are also more sensitive to the cold due to their large amount of surface area relative to their volume or body mass. Being smaller may also help dissipate extra heat helping out people living in warm areas near the equator. Getting too small may make one prone to more predators and less able to get a mate so extreme sizes are deselected. Presently heating and air conditioning systems use large amounts of our economic resources. In Britain most people heat their homes and businesses at 60F in the cold weather. British tourists get overheated easily in the USA in our warm over heated hotels and homes. For newborn or small infants room temperatures of 70 to 80F may be necessary to help them survive and grow well even when they are fully clothed but for most of us over 20 pounds temperatures of 60F will usually suffice especially when dressed warmly, eating well, and doing routine exercising that produces heat. The frail inactive elderly may also need higher temperatures to maintain their body temperature above 95F. In the USA Civil War cold stress and a poor diet accounted for many of the 2,900 deaths among 12,100 Confederate prisoners at Elmira, NY. The Southerners called it "Helmira". The camp had flimsy barracks and the winter was severe. Only those overweight on entry survived http://www.civilwarhistory.com/ElmiraPrison/Elmira.htm. The overweight became thin and the thin mostly perished. For healthy people over 20 pounds and without disabilities, such as underweight or frailty, lowering the thermostat to 60F in the cold weather will also help with weight reduction besides saving on heating bills http://www.bt.cdc.gov/disasters/winter/faq.asp. Your body uses up calories when it produces heat by muscle activity with exercise and/or shivering. Exercise equipment that generates energy is good for energy conservation, fitness, and decentralized secure energy sources. This exercise equipment may produce electric energy to be stored in batteries or use the electricity to break apart water into hydrogen and oxygen. The hydrogen may be uses in fuel cells to produce electricity or for combustion for cooking or heat. This production of energy by exercise will get you warmer and will also help give us more energy security through the decentralization of energy reserves and by reducing the demand on decreasing reserves of fossil fuels. The economic returns from the exercise will also help us to continue exercising on a regular basis for maximal benefits for our muscles, blood vessels, and heart; and by conserving scarce resources for all http://www.cdc.gov/nccdphp/dnpa/physical/index.htm. The PHIT might be used to track our exercise and our energy reserves for our individual health and our community assets. It might also help with scheduling community owned energy producing exercise equipment at convenient locations. When just needing to travel short distances we may walk or bicycle to help keep ourselves stay warm and save on the energy of moving large vehicles. In extreme weather to stay warm or cool or dry we may use the PHIT for secure and private hitchhiking, carpooling and/or bus scheduling to use our resources most efficiently.

By our daily activities we produce heat. When the environment is about as hot as or hotter than we are, then we have problems getting rid of our heat. Body temperatures over 106F may cause permanent brain damage and temperatures above 102F may sometimes cause temporary delirium. Hydration helps us to sweat or perspire to get rid of heat http://www.bt.cdc. gov/disasters/extremeheat/heat_guide.asp. In a dry climate we may fail to notice the perspiration because it evaporates without forming droplets or moisture on our skin. Only in humid weather do we notice the water coming out of skin. Humid heat is worse because the evaporation takes away more heat than just liquid perspiration on our skin. Air conditioning may be life saving especially with temperatures at 100F or above or 95F and above with high humidity. As with extreme cold, infants and the frail are more sensitive. When dressed lightly yet modestly temperatures of 80F may be well tolerated. Eating less helps to keep you cooler also. Heat is produced from digesting foods especially proteins. Eating less eventually slows your metabolism and helps reduce extra fat or adipose that helps keep heat in your body. Drinking plenty of water, for an adult 1 to 2 quarts a day, helps the body's cooling system. In the South during the USA Civil War, heat stress combined with a poor water supply caused many of the 13,000 deaths among 30,000 Union prisoners at

Andersonville, Georgia http://www.cr.nps.gov/seac/histback. htm. Taking a cool or tepid bath or shower will also help you get rid of heat. In most places the water temperature is much less than the high air temperature of the day and using some water is usually less expensive than using air conditioning. Body cooling at bedtime often helps us get to sleep. Our body temperature usually is highest at 8PM. Taking a cool bath or shower then may also help in getting to sleep. Exercise does produce heat but it also increases the thermostat setting in the brain from 98 to 99F to 100 to 101F. When our thermostat is set higher we feel more comfortable in a warm environment. Body temperatures of 101 to 104 actually help to kill off some pathogenic germs. Moderate exercise with care to avoid extreme brain damaging temperatures of 106F or more might help your comfort. Excess air conditioning to lower temperatures below 80F in hot weather may be a waste of precious energy. Sometimes rapid cooling is needed if a person's temperature is getting near 106F but otherwise being in an extra cool area much of the time prevents the body from adapting to the heat. Usually the body can adapt to weather changes in 2 to 3 days with better ability to work in a different temperature and humidity environment. Rapid changes with extreme air conditioning may be stressful with drying out of the body and chilling. Trees, parks, and grass help to get rid of some heat. Cities tend to be 5 to 10F warmer than surrounding natural areas due to the heat retained more in pavement and buildings. Plants tend to get rid of heat with natural evaporation and some conversion of sunlight into natural plant sugars or photosynthesis. Basement areas or subsurface soil tends to be cooler than the surface soil or pavement. Staying on lower floors or going into basements helps to stay cooler. Pipes carrying water through deeper soil may get rid of heat in buildings in an efficient manner. PHIT systems may help match cooler environments with people more in need of relief from heat stress. Home bound elderly may be tracked to be sure they are doing well in their particular microenvironment due to heat, cold, nutrition, exercise, or access to medication/treatment problems. If problems are found PHIT may get the community resources to them efficiently, privately and securely.

Air movements usually helps bring in oxygen and remove carbon dioxide, smoke and other toxic gasses we may produce or create. With large velocity such in tornadoes or hurricanes or shock waves with bomb blasts it may kill. Insufficient air movement may cause the sick building syndrome. The consumer health section at the National Library of Medicine (NLM) http://www.nlm.nih.gov/medlineplus/indoorairpollution. html has much information on it. Fatal forms often occur with natural disasters when people use fires or electrical generators indoors without venting thereby accumulating carbon monoxide. Low doses of carbon monoxide in smokers, car garage workers, tunnel workers, and workers around much pollution from gasoline or diesel powered internal combustion engines will speed the hardening of the arteries and lead to heart attacks. High levels of carbon dioxide may just cause headaches and sleepiness before it reaches a fatal dose. Excess air movement may cause trees and houses to collapse. The CDC lists information and resources for severe weather events http://www.bt.cdc.gov/disasters/. Building to resist such rare events may be expensive and warning systems to help get people to shelters often fail to give enough warning and avoid false warnings for tornados. We are doing fairly well with hurricanes when people have the resources to respond. Trailers are especially susceptible to wind damage but are often the only low cost housing available in rural areas. Should parts of the USA that lack such high wind events subsidize those areas that have them through disaster relief? Should industries that relocate to high-risk areas pay extra taxes or insurance? Should the northern USA be subsidized for our chronically bad winters? There are many external factors in the market value of land and labor that have environmental consequences. We really need PHIT to tracks the costs and benefits to society of locating businesses and residences in different areas of the USA and the world. Plans for different ways of using energy, varying sea levels and possible ice age scenarios would have to be factored in. We would all benefit if work and living were done most efficiently and enjoyably with market forces adjusted for social and environmental long-term values.

Breathing puts us in intimate contact with chemicals, particles, germs, dryness, humidity, heat and cold. One of these chemicals we need at least every 6 minutes or so to keep our brains, nerves, and muscles working well. Of course that is oxygen. We also must expel carbon dioxide to keep our body from getting too acidic and our brains from getting too sleepy. Our vertebrate fish ancestors first started using lungs about 160 million years ago as fish came into shallow waters then onto land http://www.sciencefriday.com/pages/2006/Apr/hour2_040706.html. Plants had to start producing oxygen and food sources on land before that occurred. Our upper respiratory system tries to filter out large particles of dust, plant matter and dirt. Smoke comes from fires in enclosed spaces such as ancient caves and in the past few hundred years in large cities with coal and wood fireplaces and stoves. Many suffered from lung disease and the combination of air pollution and germs was especially bad. Tuberculosis was the number one cause of death from the late mid 1800's to the early 1900's. Dr Edward Trudeau (Great Grandfather of Gary the cartoonist for "Doonesbury") discovered by chance that his near fatal tuberculosis got better when he left New York City and went up to Saranac Lake to Paul Smith's hunting lodge. He continued to benefit from this change in his environment and many of his patients benefited also http://www.lungusa. org/site/apps/s/content.asp?c=dvLUK9O0E&b=34706&ct=674 08 . Industrial processes have created diseases with textile fiber dust (byssinosis), asbestosis from working with insulation; and silicosis in coal workers and sand blasters and glass workers. See MedlinePlus at the NLM web site for more information on each   http://www.nlm.nih.gov/medlineplus/medlineplus.html. Of course smoking cigarettes discussed above continues to be a major cause of harm to the lungs with both toxic carcinogenic chemicals and air passage clogging particles. The dust from the World Trade Center twin towers destruction continues to harm people exposed during the 9/11 2001 attack as victims or rescuers. Chemical warfare agents may enter the lungs to destroy them, such as mustard gas or phosgene, or may enter the body through the lungs or skin then produce nerve damage, such as sarin or VX. The first poison gases were invented by Fritz Haber for the Germans in World War I to try to break the stalemate of trench warfare http://www.npr.org/templates/ story/story.php?storyId=4787312. His invention of synthetic gunpowder helped prolong the war. He also invented synthetic fertilizer that has helped feed billions of people. His chemist wife committed suicide during World War I. He was Jewish and later persecuted by the Nazi's. The poison gases were later used in concentration camps to murder Jews. He dealt with mammoth evolutionary and personal life problems. For more on chemical agents of disease see http://www.bt.cdc.gov/chemical/. A PHIT with environmental monitoring will help us detect future airborne problems. Truthful PHIT information with compassion will help us tolerate diversity in our population and benefit from its contributions to all.

Some germs by themselves may be quite toxic to the lungs. Anthrax spores specially prepared as a weapon so that they get deep into our lungs will be fatal about one half the times if untreated by antibiotics within 6 days of onset. In some high-risk areas the air is monitored for anthrax to help detect it earlier and physicians are encouraged to think about it early in an acute lung infection. Natural anthrax that occurs in cattle in the western USA usually just infects the skin and when treated heals with little long-term effect http://www.bt.cdc.gov/agent/anthrax/needtoknow.asp. An accident in a production plant in the Soviet Union showed how deadly weapon grade anthrax could be in 1979 http://www.pbs.org/wgbh/pages/frontline/shows/plague/sverdlovsk/. Flu or influenza only kills 1 to 5 % of people but infects almost all people. Pandemic flu that spreads easily in the air from person to person may affect the whole world. Pandemic flu in 1918 killed about 500,000 to 5,000,000 people in the USA out of a total of 103,000,000 people or about 0.5 to 5% of the people in the country. Besides death it incapacitated many young productive adults for about a week causing disruption in services http://www.pandemicflu.gov/general/#impact. At least some of the pandemic flu deaths were associated with air pollution as were tuberculosis deaths at the time http://www.pbs.org/wgbh/amex/influenza/peopleevents/pandeAMEX86.html. The CDC site http://www.bt.cdc.gov/agent/agentlist-category.asp lists other agents and diseases that may be used by terrorists and occur naturally. Common germs such as streptococcus, pneumococci, mycoplasma, RSV (Respiratory

Syncytial Virus) in infants, and regular influenza ("flu") all may cause severe and sometimes fatal respiratory illness. Smokers and children around smokers or others with chronic lung stress or immune problems will be affected more seriously. Newly discovered germs such as the SARS coronovirus and metapneumonia virus may cause more problems in the future. In the immunodeficient PCP (pneumocystis carinii pneumonia or pneumocystis jiroveci) may be debilitating unless the person is on an antibacterial regularly http://www.cdc.gov/ncidod/dpd/parasites/pneumocystis/default.htm. Small pox is a virus that had spread naturally and by germ warfare until 1977 when it was eliminated from natural circulation among people by the use of targeted immunization http://www.cartercenter.org/viewdoc.asp?docID=1045&submenu=news. The virus is mainly spread by the respiratory route when the patient starts coughing with smallpox pimples in their throat that occur when the smallpox rash first appears 2 to 3 days after the fever starts. It is possible to transmit the smallpox before getting the rash but it rarely occurs. It is also possible to spread small pox from the virus shed from the rash onto clothes and blankets but that is less common than spread from close respiratory contact http://www.bt.cdc.gov/agent/smallpox/disease/faq.asp. At least in Colonial America the British encouraged the spread of smallpox by giving blankets from smallpox victims to enemy American Indians http://www.nativeweb.org/pages/legal/amherst/fenn.html. George Washington was so concerned about possible deliberate spread of smallpox and the natural spread of it that he had his troops inoculated: smallpox virus from the skin pox of a sick person was scratched into the skin of a healthy person who had never had smallpox. About 2% of the people inoculated died from smallpox inoculation but that was better than the 7% of the people that died from smallpox transmitted

naturally http://en.wikipedia.org/wiki/Smallpox#ref_GWash.
In 1796 Dr. Edward Jenner demonstrated that taking cowpox
from a milkmaid and scratching that into skin of healthy
nonimmune people would protect them from smallpox. This
was called vaccination. This had much less hazard than the
inoculation procedure. In 1972 in the USA we stopped using
smallpox vaccination since the disease was so rare that the side
effects became more of a problem than the disease. About 1 in
1000 might get a severe eye or skin infection with eczema, and
1 in 10,000 might die of complications especially if they had
immunodeficiency. This would have been worth the risk if we
were still having epidemics with 7% of the population dying
but with control of the disease in the USA and in travelers we
were able to avoid it. With smallpox we are also able to vaccinate
contacts to prevent disease. This has to occur within 3 days of
exposure to the disease but it is effective http://www.bt.cdc.gov/
agent/smallpox/vaccination/faq.asp. In 2003 we revaccinated
some health care workers so that they might respond with
little risk to any possible cases of smallpox from bioterrorism.
With or without terrorists new germs may emerge. In 1977 an
outbreak of pneumonia at a Veteran's meeting in Philadelphia,
Pennsylvania came from an air conditioner contaminated with
bacteria that had previously been unknown though treated
with tetracycline or erythromycin http://www.cdc.gov/ncidod/
dbmd/diseaseinfo/legionellosis_g.htm. For protection from
germs, toxins and particulates respirators are helpful when
used correctly. N-95 masks and APR (air-purifying respirators)
might be used more in high-risk situations http://www.cdc.
gov/niosh/docs/2005-100/chapter2.html#chapt2b.   Simple
droplet stopping facemasks are used commonly in Asia but
USA experts doubt their value. In the USA we emphasize
hand washing by all, and isolation of contagious people. In

the future new germs such as pandemic influenza, legionella, SARS, and metapneumonia virus will continue to emerge and a PHIT should be ready to detect, control and if possible treat them in the manner most appropriate for the particular germ.

Eating is a way that we interact intimately with the chemicals in the environment. We digest some with acids and enzymes but some remain unchanged and enter our blood stream. Natural toxins from staphylococcus germs that are heat resistant may make us vomit, cough and get warm. Staphylococcus grows well on ham and cold cuts and pudding http://www.cdc.gov/ncidod/dbmd/diseaseinfo/staphylococcus_food_g.htm#7. This toxin might be used by poisoning foods or drink. This toxin is resistant to heat. Clostridium botulinum grows from spores easily and grows well in canned or anaerobic environments producing a toxin resistant to heat below 140F or 70C. The toxin causes muscle weakness with double vision being an early sign. It may also be used to poison food or drink. In babies fed honey containing its spores the germ may grow in the intestines causing constipation and muscle weakness http://www.bt.cdc.gov/agent/botulism/index.asp. The toxin is used to loosen muscles that are too tight or in spasm in the preparation known as BOTOX. In large amounts the muscle weakness leads to death by asphyxiation when the muscles that expand and contract our lungs stop working. Anthrax discussed above may also be ingested, then cause bloody diarrhea and fever. Every winter and spring in the USA rotavirus spreads from the southwest part of the country to the northeast with often severe vomiting and diarrhea experienced by infants and toddlers. People may get the virus repeatedly but the first time usually gives the worst symptoms. A vaccine for infants was used in 1998 then discontinued due to an increased incidence of intussusception http://www.cdc.gov/ncidod/dvrd/revb/ gastro/rotavirus.htm. A new vaccine without this complication is now available http://www.cdc.gov/nip/diseases/rota/rota-faqs. htm#vaccine. Rotavirus now causes 400,000 doctor's visits and 50,000 hospitalizations with costs of $1 billion per year; and 5-10% of all diarrhea and 50% of all hospitalization for diarrhea for children less than 5 years old. Noroviruses often cause outbreaks on cruise ships and in gatherings of people if food or surfaces get contaminated from sick people http:// www.cdc.gov/ncidod/dvrd/revb/gastro/norovirus-qa.htm. Shigellosis is a bacterial form of diarrhea spread mostly among preschoolers and their families. Salmonella Typhi may cause severe gastroenteritis with blood stream infection and Typhoid Fever but only 400 cases occur in the USA now. Travelers to developing countries are at increased risk. They should get vaccinated and avoid raw unpeeled foods http://www.cdc. gov/ncidod/dbmd/diseaseinfo/typhoidfever_g.htm. Other salmonella strains, toxic e coli, and campylobacter infections are common in chicken and cattle. Poultry and meats should be cooked and raw drippings should be cleaned from any raw food processing areas and raw food handlers. Some people may get arthritis after salmonella or campylobacter infections. A rare but severe nerve disease with weakness of the legs called Guillain-Barre Syndrome may occur after campylobacter infections http://www.cdc.gov/az.do#N. Listeria is a bacterium present in many animals and often contaminating cold cuts and hot dogs. It may be especially dangerous in pregnant women, newborns, and the immunosuppressed. Cryptosporidium and giardia are parasites that live in cattle and many wild animals. They are resistant to chlorination but municipal water treatment filters will usually remove them. Young children, pregnant women and immunosuppressed people should be especially careful

http://www.cdc.gov/ncidod/dpd/parasites/cryptosporidiosis/default.htm http://www.cdc.gov/ncidod/dpd/parasites/giardiasis/default.htm . There are many other known germs that may cause many illnesses but all may be prevented with good quality sanitation, water and food. The most common salmonella germs, toxic e coli, campylobacter, and Listeria may all be greatly reduced by adopting a whole food plant derived diet. Sometimes toxic e coli may contaminate vegetables such as spinach but usually it is derived from nearby farm animals.

For the unknown we need PHIT or other accessible yet private and secure information on what we are eating and how healthy we are. In 1989 a new Syndrome: Eosinophilia-Myalgia appeared. It was linked to a change in the production of a nutritional supplement: L-tryptophan http://www.emedicine.com/med/topic693.htm. The Mad Cow Disease or Bovine Spongiform Encephalopathy (BSE) came from a change in feeding cattle that cause a severe brain illness in a few people 10 years later. Without good records and statistics it would have been hard to detect. Now we avoid feeding cows and other animals any body parts from cows to avoid passing prions to any other animals http://www.cdc.gov/ncidod/dvrd/bse/. A well maintained PHIT should help us catch any future food borne illness caused by changes in technology or criminal behavior: genetic modification, antibiotic use, pesticides, herbicides, production, chemical additives etc.

Before leaving the realm of germs, we should note that most intestinal germs are helpful to us. They live in our intestines and produce vitamin K necessary for our normal clotting mechanisms. Lactobacillus acidophilus may be taken in supplements http://www.nlm.nih.gov/medlineplus/druginfo/natural/patient-acidophilus.html. It helps prevent vaginal yeast infections and on further study may be useful for controlling yeast, cholesterol and allergies http://www.mayoclinic.com/health/probiotics/AN00389, and http://en.wikipedia.org/wiki/Probiotics. Recently researchers have found that whipworm parasites that may live in our intestines produce chemicals that decrease inflammation. This makes it easier for the whipworms to survive in our intestines by decreasing our immune response to the worms and also relieves diseases caused by inflammation http://apnews.excite.com/article/20060610/D8I51RHO0.html. Using pig whipworms in humans in the future might be a way to help people with Crohn's Disease and Ulcerative Colitis. If we avoid the parasites and germs especially toxic to humans, organic foods naturally enriched with a healthy mix of micro flora and micro flora might help keep our immune system in balance.

Just being natural fails to guarantee that it is healthy. Many natural chemicals in foods are toxic. We all know to avoid poison mushrooms that look quite similar to regular mushrooms. Cooked mushrooms have fewer carcinogens than raw mushrooms but cooking fails to eliminate toxins from poisonous mushrooms http://calpoison.org/public/mushrooms.html. Some species are now developing new toxins http://www.foxnews.com/story/0,2933,207133,00.html. Moldy peanuts contain aflatoxin that causes liver cancer, shellfish grown in red tide causes food poisoning etc. http://vm.cfsan.fda.gov/~mow/intro.html for a complete listing of common germ and chemical problems in food. Colin Campbell notes that children and rats on low animal protein diets rarely get cancer from aflatoxin http://www.thechinastudy.com/. Lately a toxin from eating cycad plants has been shown to possibly cause ALS (Amyotrophic Lateral Sclerosis) or Lou Gehrig's disease in Guam http://www.npr.org/templates/story/story.

php?storyId=1500851 audio story, http://www.ncbi.nlm.nih. gov/entrez/query.fcgi?cmd=Retrieve&db=pubmed&dopt=A bstract&list_uids=16008818&query_hl=1&itool=pubmed_ docsum abstract at NLM, cycad information http://plantnet. rbgsyd.gov.au/PlantNet/cycad/toxic.html . The indigenous people on Guam have a high incidence of ALS and other neurological diseases likely caused from eating flour or pollen or bats that ingest the pollen from the cycad plants. Some of the same natural chemicals have been found in North Americans with ALS but the source of the chemicals in North America is as of yet unknown. For us omnivore's we must continually evaluate our food source safety and the outcomes of eating different foods with the help of PHIT.

Close contacts with other organisms or their secretions that carry germs may transmit biohazards. In the Sexually Transmitted Infection Chapter we discussed the risks from germs from other people and their blood and body fluids. Here we will discuss some common germs that live in other species. In the USA we are fortunate at present to be free of any major germs from other species. West Nile Virus (WNV), Eastern Equine Encephalitis; parasites in cat, dog, and raccoon feces; worms in meats, rabies, plague and many other animal viruses may occasionally infect us by mosquito transmission, animal bite, flea bite, poor sanitation from dirty hands or children putting their fingers in their mouths, or by eating of poorly cooked meat. In the developing world malaria, schistosomiasis, filariasis and leishmaniasis are frequent causes of disability and death. Malaria is transmitted by mosquitoes and causes about 1 million deaths per year http://www.cdc.gov/malaria/ . Schistosomiasis is carried by freshwater snails and is caused by bathing in or drinking water with the parasite. About 120 million are ill and 20 million disabled from schistosomiasis or bilharzias caused by microscopic worms http://www.cdc.gov/ ncidod/dpd/parasites/schistosomiasis/default.htm, http://www. emedicine.com/emerg/topic857.htm. Filariasis is transmitted by mosquito and infects about 120 million people in the world causing swollen lymph nodes, arms and legs http://www.cdc. gov/ncidod/dpd/parasites/lymphaticfilariasis/default.htm. Leishmaniasis is transmitted by sand flies with 1.5 million new cases of skin or cutaneous infections and 0.5 million of visceral or inner organ infections each year in the world http://www.cdc. gov/ncidod/dpd/parasites/leishmania/factsht_leishmania.htm . These are just the well-known problems. With global climate change diseases may come and go with changing distribution of host animals and the vectors such as mosquitoes, fleas, and sand flies that transmit the diseases. Germs that now may just bother animals may get into people as we move into new territories or animals such as migrating birds move into new territories. Eating a whole food plant derived diet will help eliminate many of the animal carried germs. Again real time online private and secure PHIT systems are needed throughout our world to tract diseases, vectors, host animals, treatments, preventive techniques and their outcomes.

CHAPTER 11
Fat Wars: DHA and Vitamin D versus Trans Saturated Fats with Sugar

Trans-fatty acids fight to clog and inflame our arteries while DHA and HDL defend our arteries and active Vitamin D decreases inflammation, autoimmune disease and cancer. The quality of fats in our body makes a big difference. Trans-fats or hydrogenated fats tend to reduce the HDL (high density lipoproteins) in our blood stream. The HDL acts as an antioxidant that helps to keep the walls of the arteries clean and free flowing http://www.umm.edu/features/transfats.html. Good blood supply to our brains, heart muscles, kidneys and skeletal muscles are crucial to our body's functions. In 2002 the National Academy of Science's Institute of Medicine recommended that manufactured or added trans saturated fats be eliminated from our diets http://www.iom.edu/CMS/5410.aspx. So far Congress and the FDA (Food and Drug Administration) have just required the labeling of the trans-fats content of packaged foods. Now on food labels in the USA the trans-fats line shows the number of grams of trans-saturated fats in a serving of that food. If the amount is less than 0.5 grams then the label may state zero. Since low levels still may cause harm for susceptible individuals you may avoid trans-saturated fats completely by making sure that the ingredient list lacks partially hydrogenated fats or vegetable shortening or margarine. We now have so much trans-fat in our diet because a German chemist Wilhelm Normann found an inexpensive way to produce a tasty semi-solid fat from soy oil that kept well http://en.wikipedia.org/wiki/Trans_fat. People unaware of its long term consequences for heart problems, and aware of its cheaper price and better shelf life, used it in place of lard or compound lard that had come into common use in the 1800's http://www.fengshuitours.com/sfc/MSPproducts511. asp. It still tastes good, is cheap and keeps well; so many fast food restaurants, franchises and food manufacturers are finding it hard to replace. A popular replacement that avoids the trans-fat problem creates problems with regular saturated fats and the environment. Palm oil is a saturated fat that will increase our cholesterol levels. For most people this will increase our LDL (low density lipoprotein) cholesterol and increase our heart disease risk from increased clogging of our arteries. Since palm oil is free of trans-fat at least it will fail to decrease our good HDL. If we exercise enough, stay slim, and take in much oat bran with soluble fiber to suck the cholesterol out of our intestines and body, then it harm our body little. It may have a large impact on our world's endangered ecosystems and species by replacing rain forests with palm oil plantations http://www. cspinet.org/palm/. As I write these changes in diet, exercise, and environment are occurring. What will be there net effect? Will we have to wait for a new epidemic of chronic disease or an environmental catastrophe to know? We should be informing concerned humans and monitoring these changes as they occur with PHIT.

In order to help protect our arteries, besides staying trim and exercising; taking some DHA (docosahexaenoic acid), EPA (eicosapentaenoic acid) and Vitamin D will likely help. About 1 to 2 grams of fish oil containing DHA and EPA (omega 3 fatty acids) helps reduce triglycerides in our blood and helps make with the cell membranes in our blood vessels and brains. It also helps with blood pressure and Rheumatoid Arthritis, and likely helps brain development in babies and mental test results in the elderly pending further study http://www.nlm.nih.gov/medlineplus/druginfo/natural/patient-fishoil.html, http://www.umm.edu/altmed/ConsSupplements/DocosahexaenoicAcidDHAcs.html .We have to avoid eating more than one serving per week of white tuna, tilefish, swordfish, or halibut because of mercury toxicity. Eating animals low on the food chain like sardines or scallops or shrimp is safer because they contain less mercury. Pregnant and nursing women should be even more careful by eating no more than one serving of mercury containing fish a month since developing fetuses and babies have more sensitive brains http://en.wikipedia.org/wiki/Minamata_disease. Fish oil supplements are available now at most drug or nutrition stores. The supplements made from distilled fish oil usually have low safe levels of mercury and PCB (poly chlorinated biphenyls) even though these are found in undistilled big fish oil. The fish oil is usually gotten from small fish that often are the food for feeding bigger fish in the ocean or on fish farms or wild shore birds. This may cause some undesirable environmental changes. There is also DHA made from genetically modified algae. This is theoretically safer if done right and is now the source of the DHA that is put in baby formulas and marketed to pregnant women and breast-feeding mothers (with one brand named Expecta in the USA). This brand is more expensive than the fish oil now but as fish become scarcer and algae production becomes better it will likely become a better source. Algae may be dangerous if grown incorrectly because they may produce toxins under certain conditions http://www.cfsan.fda.gov/~mow/chap37.html. Soybeans, walnuts, flax seed and other plants provide alpha-linolenic acid (ALA) that may be

made into EPA then DHA in small amounts in humans http://
en.wikipedia.org/wiki/Alpha-linolenic_acid. New genetically
engineered soybeans made to make better frying oil will have
little ALA.

Vitamin D besides helping us absorb and use calcium for
our bones also helps our muscles, pancreas and blood pressure.
Vitamin D is fat-soluble so may be stored in our body. From
May to September in the Northern Hemisphere north of San
Diego and Florida the sun is strong enough to give us a week's
supply from about 2 hours of skin exposure but from October
to April the sun is too weak to give much Vitamin D even with
prolonged exposure in this area. Vitamin D is added to milk
so that drinking 4 cups (1 quart or liter) of milk will give us
an adequate amount for a child or 200 units (5 mcg) of it but
now many experts recommend 400 to 800 units per day. Colin
Campbell recommends that we avoid milk for its possible cancer
and heart disease promoting effects. Most multivitamins for
adults have 400 units. One study showed that children given
extra Vitamin D had a lower incidence of diabetes mellitus of
the Type I or Juvenile or Insulin Dependent kind. People with
Type II diabetes become more sensitive to the insulin when
given Vitamin D in preliminary studies that need further
confirmation http://www.nlm.nih.gov/medlineplus/druginfo/
natural/patient-vitamind.html. Complicating the Vitamin D
studies is the need to analyze the amount of animal protein
and calcium in the diet. Colin Campbell points out that diets
high in animal protein and calcium tend to decrease the
biologically active form of Vitamin D (1, 25 hydroxy Vitamin
D) http://www.thechinastudy.com/. Preventing and controlling
diabetes mellitus is important to help keep arteries clean and
open. When we have higher blood sugar or glucose levels the

small artery wall get thicker blocking blood flow. The large arteries get more plaque or hardened growths inside the arteries due to the LDL that is glycalated. With diabetes the glucose chemically bonds to the LDL making it more potent in producing intra-arterial plaques. With insulin resistance higher insulin levels are needed and that increases the LDL and triglycerides in the blood stream making the plaque creation problem even worse. With so many factors in constant flux we need PHIT to make any sense out of this and help to inform everyone of what is really known. Once again note that more exercise and less calorie consumption help too.

CHAPTER 12
Genes: A Natural Information System

Our DNA (deoxyribonucleic acid) encodes instructions to build and run our body. The information is encoded in the pattern of 4 nucleic acids paired with another nucleic acid arranged in the double helix. The Human Genome Project has discovered the pattern of the 3 billion base pairs but we still must figure out what it means. We believe there are about 24,000 to 30,000 genes within these 3 billion base pairs http://www.ornl.gov/sci/techresources/Human_Genome/faq/genenumber.shtml. [This is like knowing all the letters and their order a book but we still need to learn the words, sentences and paragraphs to give the book meaning.] A gene is a section of the sequence of these base pairs that codes for creation of one protein that helps in the function of the cell. We do know 6,000 single gene disorders but for most other genes we need to find out what they are and what they do http://www.ornl.gov/sci/techresources/Human_Genome/medicine/assist.shtml . Most of the DNA resides on 23 pairs of chromosomes in the nucleus of our cells. In the male one pair of chromosomes is unequal with an X and Y chromosome; otherwise we usually have one each of chromosomes and thus one of each gene from each parent. Only males carry the Y chromosome. The Y chromosome is smaller and has fewer genes than the X chromosome. Some genes only reside on the X chromosome such as the Hemophilia A gene and therefore males will only have one copy of a gene that is only on the X chromosome. Some DNA also resides in the mitochondria in each cell in our body. The mitochondrial DNA comes from the egg cell, thus we only get one copy of this DNA and it comes from our biologic mother. We know that have 3 copies of a chromosome such as number 21 gives Down syndrome. Why would an extra normal chromosome give us problems? We are still working on that. Some individuals have an abnormal gene for diseases such as Tuberous Sclerosis or Neurofibromatosis and do well but other family members may have catastrophic medical problems with the same gene. Histones are proteins associated with our DNA that may regulate when and how genes function or become expressed http://en.wikipedia.org/wiki/Histone. For a more detailed introduction to medical genetics see the Children's Hospital of Philadelphia web site: http://www.chop. edu/consumer/your_child/module_toc.jsp?id=-8537.

A large impetus to develop better public health information technology (PHIT) is the possibility in the near future of being inundated with huge amounts of information about our most important genes. This is also a motivation to be sure that our PHIT is private and secure yet helpful to individuals and their designated health care providers. For years we have screened newborns for PKU (phenylketonuria), thyroid deficiency and sickle cell disease. When these problems are found immediate intervention helps prevent the infant from developing permanent disability. With PKU we change the infant's diet, with thyroid deficiency we give thyroid medication to the infant, and with sickle cell disease we closely monitor the child for infections and clotting problems. The health departments or screening companies keep the information confidential so that only the infant's family and health care providers know the infant's problems. Newborn screening started in 1965 with the work of Dr. Robert Guthrie at the University of

Buffalo http://www.pku-allieddisorders.org/guthrie.htm. He developed the science and technology and went on to crusade for its implementation to help prevent mental retardation. Finding the disease in his niece and help from his colleagues at Buffalo inspired him. Now in NY State we screen for 40 different conditions in newborns http://www.wadsworth. org/newborn/index.htm. NY State has an electronic database and tracking system but it lacks easy access by the families of newborns and their doctors. For more information on newborn screening see the NLM MedlinePlus site http://www.nlm. nih.gov/medlineplus/newbornscreening.html. Now mail and phone contacts are required to follow up on possibly significant results. With more tests being done there will be more true and false positive results and some results important to the next generation. When testing for sickle cell disease or cystic fibrosis now the laboratory often finds newborns with just one gene for the disease. For most genes we have duplicate copies. For autosomal recessive diseases like sickle cell disease or cystic fibrosis we need 2 copies of a defective gene to get the disease. When we just have one defective gene and one good gene we usually lack any apparent symptoms. Sometimes having one copy of a defective gene is actually helpful. With sickle trait or the people with just one gene for sickle cell they seem to have some resistance to severe malarial infections. With cystic fibrosis the carriers with the one defective gene may be able to have more children than non-carriers. These advantages for the carrier state help perpetuate some of these potentially harmful but usually helpful genes in the population. The disease state with the 2 defective genes might be prevented if the mating of carriers for the same gene defect is discouraged. This has been done for years in the conservative Hasidic Jewish communities where matchmakers are given information on Tay—Sachs disease gene carriers who are common in this population and then advise against any matches between two carriers. This has worked with some success. For more information on this and other genetic diseases see the Online Mendelian Inheritance in Man (OMIM) site at the National Library of Medicine. It is up to date and authoritative http://www.ncbi.nlm.nih.gov/entrez/query.fcgi?db=OMIM&itool=toolbar. The site is based on the life long work of Dr. Victor A. McKusick from Maine and then a Professor at Johns Hopkins University School of Medicine who helped create the medical specialty of genetics. He was inspired as a youth by the Jumping Frenchman of Maine phenomena described at the OMIM web site.

For the general population in the future data from current family histories, newborn screening and future DNA biochip screening analysis will allow singles to check for possible genetic problems before they date someone. Biochips that detect DNA or genes with problems are predicted to be a relatively inexpensive way to screen for 50 to 150 genes, on a signal test chip. Screening may be done for genes that may cause significant health problems such as Factor V Leiden. This gene predisposes to clotting that causes deep vein clots with emboli or pulmonary embolisms. This gene occurs in about 3% of Caucasians. Women that have Factor V Leiden on birth control pills have a much greater risk of clotting. Men or women with it when forced to rest such as on long trips or after surgery have more risks for clotting or thrombosis. The State or some well-regulated independent agency may check a database of the results of genetic testing and/or family history for each potential mating pair. The information might interface in a confidential way with current dating services or dating web sites or a free secure service to registered users with a forge proof machine readable identity card with PIN (personal identity number) and/or bioidentifier such as a finger print, face scan or iris scan. The individuals involved would be told that the match would have a high biologic risk for any progeny but information on any specifics would be kept from other people and if desired the information may be kept from the individual themselves. The individual or the family of a child would decide who would get information on recessive genes or tendencies that lack any immediate known health consequences. If future information shows likely health consequences then the health care providers currently involved with the patient would be informed through the PHIT and the information would be discussed with the patient to the extent desired by the patient and/or their custodian. For couples that have already formed a social pairing genetic information may be used to discuss possible risks for their progeny and possible ways to avoid them such as adoption, or in vitro fertilization with genetic testing of the fertilized eggs before implanting them into the mother's womb, or planning for a genetic problem that might be treated early before a permanent problem occurred such as with PKU disease. The public health issues surrounding genetics and the interaction with the environment are further discussed at http://www.cdc.gov/node.do/id/0900f3ec8000e2b5. The CDC is also encouraging the technically simple creation of family histories to help detect significant genetic and/or environmental problems to watch for. These potentially problems may be discussed and worked on at a preconception medical visit also recommended by the CDC http://www.cdc.gov/ncbddd/preconception/default.htm. One of the key roles of PHIT will be to fully define the effect of genes on our health throughout our lives and how they interact with our environment, nutrition, medications and health care. With so many possibly important genes, so many gene-to-gene interactions, and so many environmental variables; a PHIT well integrated with our EHR's (Electronic Health Records) is needed for interventions and study with CQI (Continuing Quality Improvement) and economic evaluation to help determine what of many things we should do first. Only with PHIT will the meaning of the Human Genome Project to our day-to-day existence and our future be found.

Now we should discuss if people in overcrowded areas, young teenagers, mental incompetents, abusive individuals and violent criminals should be discouraged from having children. Due to the abuse of minorities with discriminatory sterilizations, ethnic cleansing, genocide, and the problem of determining who will be the best parents and what traits will help our species in the unknown future, society and courts are loathe enter into this complex fray http://en.wikipedia.org/wiki/ Eugenics . Fortunately people will refrain from child bearing when economic conditions are poor as in the 1930's depression years and when educated and social supports beyond families exist. In the developing world educating females usually leads to a decreased birth rate in most countries http://www.prb. org/Publications/PolicyBriefs/EmpoweringWomenDevelopi ngSocietyFemaleEducationintheMiddleEastandNorthAfrica. aspx . When the government provides a safety net such as social security families usually have less children. In a purely agrarian economy many children help with the farm work and chores and help to care for the elderly http://en.wikipedia.org/ wiki/Population. China tried to decrease their birth rate with rewards for families with just one child but it was unpopular and the effect of education and economic development likely helped more than their policy http://www.overpopulation. com/faq/Population_Control/one_child.html. Singapore also tried to decrease their growth rate in the 1970's and 80's with more success than they wanted (http://lcweb2.loc.gov/frd/cs/sgtoc.html and search for population policy). As in China the education of women and the improved social environment probably helped reduce the birth rate more than the government policy. In the USA improved self-esteem in teenagers with educational or other achievements helps to decrease teen pregnancy and behavioral problem rates. Young teenagers are often biologically able to have children but in the developed world and in the technologically advancing developing world they usually lack the intellectual and occupational strengths and skills to be supportive and adaptive parents. Some community programs do help http://www.modelprograms.samhsa.gov/model.htm. In the future community service corps might also be used http://www.frankschaeffer.net/awol.html. The technology exists now to prevent pregnancies in women with injections every 3 months (Depo-Provera) or slow release hormones implanted every 3 to 5 years (Jadelle in Europe now and Norplant in the USA in the past) http://en.wikipedia.org/wiki/Birth control. To avoid anxiety about minority or individual persecution for inconsequential traits and promote diversity, we should avoid using physical coercion and continue to encourage self-esteem, education and alternatives to child bearing in our young people to help avoid problems with child rearing and overpopulation and avoid micromanaging social and biologic relationships when the logic is uncertain.

In the future we must avoid forcing our species into a narrow band of form and abilities that may lead to easy extinction. The eugenics of the late 1800's and early 1900's in the USA and in Hitler's Germany of the 1930's had many problems http://en.wikipedia.org/wiki/Eugenics. Prejudice was substituted for science. With the motivation of territorial defense and mate guarding, diversity was taken as undesirable. Present day prohibitions on same sex marriage may also be seen as mate guarding. In Germany traditional ethnic competition for territory masqueraded as social science. In the USA at the Oneida Community the elders got their pick of the young women using eugenics to justify their emotional mate guarding tendencies to dismay of the young man of the Community http://www.nyhistory.com/central/oneida.htm. This was a major reason for the break up of the Community. Sterilization was forced on 60,000 people at the beginning to the mid 1900's in the USA with eugenics often lending the respectability of science to ethnic prejudice. In Germany euthanasia was practiced on ethnic groups and the disabled. We should recognize the costs of disability and real genetic problems, then deal with it humanely taking advantage of the various abilities of all who may contribute to society. I will briefly present scenarios of possible futures that might take advantageous of genetic characteristics that are now detriments.

Presently we have an epidemic of obesity with increased in illness and costs http://www.cdc.gov/nccdphp/dnpa/obesity/. Overweight people have a high risk of diabetes, high blood pressure and heart disease. We must pay more for health care costs and they have decreased productivity due to their weight and possible illnesses. We might encourage the breeding of thin people and discourage the breeding of overweight people, however if we were struck by famine or other food supply disaster our species would be unable to survive more than a few months. An adult 100 to 200 pounds overweight may survive 2 to 4 years off the extra fat or adipose tissue. With the appropriate exercise equipment they might convert their energy into electricity to run essential equipment or to produce hydrogen from water by hydrolysis. Many people believe that is why we are able to get overweight easily. As we developed as a species only those who had gained weight easily and retained it survived early periods of famine or drought. Certainly the Indians of the southwest of the USA over the past 2 thousand years experienced regular drought and have a high incidence of diabetes mellitus.

Presently we have about 1 in 400 children with Autism. They require special schooling and supervision often http://www.cdc.gov/ncbddd/autism/. Some Autism is familial and about one third with a known genetic factor. Autistic children and adults often relate to machines better than non-Autistic children. Their problem is usually in relating to people in social relations. If we develop into a society run by computers their ability to deal with machines may be very important for our survival. Some of our best scientists and technicians have some deficits in social interactions that have directed them into the more objective studies.

In the temperate areas of the globe dark skin makes it harder to get Vitamin D and often is the target of ethnic prejudice and territoriality. If we continue to get less ozone dark skin will help to reduce the risk of sunburn and skin cancer. Taking a multivitamin tablet will get you enough Vitamin D even with dark skin. A show on NPR discusses "the melanin hypothesis". This hypothesis suggests increased melanin shows better biologic resilience http://www.npr.org/templates/story/story.php?storyId=5401182. This program also discusses how the public perceives and deals with genetics and science in general. Of course some people are better at some things than other people. Genetics plays a part in this. For the survival of our species all special capabilities, skills and talents should be valued for the increased adaptability of our species.

At present technology and computer use help in gaining more resources for the technology workers and their dependents, but with huge amounts of radioactive nuclear materials in the world the possibility of a nuclear winter is real. In that case if we survive the initial radiation surge, we would need our old primitive hunter and gather skills with strong work group coordination skills. Discouraging sports, hunting, foraging and basic agriculture might make sense in getting more high tech jobs but would be counterproductive in many possible post global disaster scenarios.

What chemicals, nerves, muscles, bones, and metabolism will help us survive in other planets in our solar system or in our galaxy? It sure is hard to tell. We should continue to prize diversity because it may save our species. Our human compassion for the weak and dependent that often appears to conservative and territorial individuals to be a waste of resources may actually be a wise investment in species adaptability.

Especially now with genetic engineering for plants and animals progressing much more rapidly than in humans we must consider keeping diversity in our ecosystems in order to allow our environment to adapt to climate and pollution changes. Man is the most invasive species who is stressing our world to its limits in many places. We must avoid species elimination and ecosystem destruction to save our species even though it may appear sentimental and irrational in light of huge short term economic gains that rapid exploitation of resources may bring. We need to appreciate the importance of long-term investments and avoid focusing solely on quarterly or yearly profits.

To help address all these issues and balance the long term and short term needs we need PHIT to evaluate getting the largest potential benefits with the minimum amount of resources. Even if we desired we are unable to keep alive for years in good condition all possible biologic variations of humans. Many are fatal within a year or two such as Trisomy 13 http://ghr.nlm.nih.gov/condition=trisomy13 and Trisomy 18 http://ghr.nlm.nih.gov/condition=trisomy18 ; but we should avoid spending resources in eliminating diversity that is able to exist without assistance. How much energy should we devote to avoiding rare though catastrophic scenarios such as the nuclear winter or the take over of our civilization by machines? How much should we spend now on water and environmental protection for developing countries? Investing in the developing world to protect their ecosystems and benefit their people would do much to help the developed world in dealing with immigration and foreign relations but the populations of the developed world need to understand this before politicians may give away their resources. The PHIT systems with privacy and security may help educate, get feed back from our populations, and continually evaluate our interventions for environmental and social health throughout the world.

CHAPTER 13
Medical Care: You Can't Live With It and You Can't Live Without It

As a technical service that helps us extend our species realm of existence, medical care will usually allow us to ascend to new heights in extracting resources from the environment, but when it fails we fall through its net of safety to the hard unforgiving ground of disability, disease and death. Medical care is part of the coping mechanism of our species to deal with our natural limitations from difficult environments, rival species and other humans. Our genes, our religion, our culture and our technical specialists try to create our best match to our changing environment to adapt, survive and reproduce. Often we fail, then medical care tries to correct for the problems. For the ancient Egyptians medical care dealt with injuries from construction to build their nation and warfare to protect it from invaders and to conquer rich territories; with anxiety caused by infections and disease through chants and magic wands; and with antibacterial herbs and minerals http://www.metmuseum.org/special/Art Medicine Egypt/medicine more.asp. Since then we have tried to accumulate more information about how our body works and how to cure or assist the body. Still we have gaps in knowledge and technology, so that the expectations of medicine as a nurturer, helper or rescuer may lead to disappointment and regret. The resulting impediment, economic damage, pain or malpractice may lead to legal case to compensate for the undisclosed or preventable complications, errors or failures in medical care. Our high expectations, often fueled by physicians themselves, lead to the feeling that physicians have failed. When patients or their families believe that physicians could have done better, we often end up in court, even though the science and technology to help in that particular case may only theoretically be possible http://en.wikipedia.org/wiki/Medical_malpractice. Specialist physicians in the 1840's who had skills and knowledge in certain areas that were better than the skills and knowledge of general practitioners in that area began to publicize this to the community and patients. Patients with serious complicated problems then went to the specialists with an expectation to be cured and some were disappointed even though their care was better than what they might have gotten elsewhere. Attorneys funded with contingency fees, sympathetic juries, malpractice insurance companies, continuing technical advances, and tort law have all contributed to this escalating expensive phenomena of medical malpractice as described in JAMA http://www.ncbi.nlm.nih.gov/entrez/query.fcgi?cmd=Retrieve&db=pubmed&dopt=Abstract&list_uids=10755500&query_hl=5&itool=pubmed_docsum. Even with the best care available in our world some diseases fail to yield to our science and technology. Physicians must try to give hope and attempt to cure difficult problems yet be realistic with patients and families on the chances of improvements and the complications and costs of the intervention. This is a difficult challenge fraught with risks of under treatment, over treatment, misunderstanding, and liability. This basically is an information problem that we often fail to address. We need information on what is the best care for the patient based on previous studies of similar patients and basic biologic information. This has to be communicated to the patient in an understandable manner and this all has to be documented. The attorneys, juries, and judges need information to evaluate what is realistically possible based on high quality research. Philip Howard, an attorney that founded Common Good, suggests that we use medical courts to help create and develop judges with medical knowledge http://cgood.org/index.html. Of course to try deal with unresponsive diseases we need continuing information on basic science, clinical trials and current patient responses to experimental treatments. Now physicians often practice based on tradition or customs, patients often only hear what they want to hear, and patients with poor outcomes go to court regardless of the quality of medical care. I will now discuss some examples of information problems in medical care and how they were solved or may be solved.

In the 1940's premature newborns were noted to often get blindness from thickening of the back of the eye or retina. This condition was called Retrolental Fibroplasia of the Newborn (RLF). Prior to the 1940's special hospital care for the newborns was rare. My grandfather, Isaac Newton and many other premature small babies were kept warm wrapped up in low heat ovens or in drawers to help their survival based on experience, folklore, and/or medical tradition. In the late 1800's and early 1900's some premature babies in incubators were shown at fairs or exhibitions to raise money for their care and inform the curious public. In the 1940's they started to notice babies were struggling to breathe so they used the new technology of oxygen supplementation then. At first it was hard to measure how much oxygen they were getting since machines or gauges to measure oxygen concentrations were unavailable. It was also very hard to know how much oxygen was getting into the blood stream of the babies from their lungs since it took large amounts of blood to check the oxygen levels. Premature babies have little blood and small veins and arteries. Some studies in some nurseries showed that babies that got more oxygen had more RLF but other studies failed to find such an association. Later it was found out that even though some babies had the same flow of oxygen going into their incubators they were getting less oxygen because of leaks in some incubators. Some babies got the same amount of oxygen in the air going into their lungs but had less oxygen in their blood stream due to worse lung disease. In later years it was found out that babies that were over 32 weeks of gestation or 32 weeks in the womb before birth were much less likely to get RLF even though they might be very small and get much oxygen. All these factors unknown to the physician pediatric specialists or neonatologists taking care of these babies made it difficult to inform the families of the patients to help them decide what to do. In the 1950's when it looked like oxygen was causing blindness from the RLF some physicians decreased the amount of oxygen that babies were getting. This did help reduce the RLF but increased other problems such as brain and kidney damage. Eventually by the 1970's the technology to more easily measure the oxygen that babies got to breath, and the amount that was in their blood stream became available, then safe levels of oxygen that were high enough to keep the brains and kidneys in shape but low enough to protect the retina were found. Through this time neonatologists continued to try to evaluate the medical care with biologic and clinical research and the outcomes of clinical research trials with eventual success. Until the information was adequate some babies got RLF but had good brains and some had good eyes but brain damage. Without any oxygen at all many of the babies would have died from respiratory failure with fatal brain and kidney damage. Physicians strived to help but unexpected side effects occurred. The good physicians noted these and studied them trying to learn from this information failure. The medical care system was cured with improved information. For a complete recounting of this story from a heroic pioneer in the field see http://www.neonatology.org/classics/parable/default.html by William A. Silverman, MD. The problem was bad but would have been tragic if physicians had failed to question the virtue of their therapies and evaluate alternate interventions that were also flawed.

In the 1970's SIDS (Sudden Infant Death Syndrome) or Crib Death occurred in 1 in 500 babies in the USA. At that time physicians recommended that babies sleep in their stomachs or face down. A young physician from the Netherlands came to the USA to do a residency in pediatrics. He took the information about sleep position back with him to the Netherlands and advised his patients' families and his colleagues that all babies should sleep on their stomach. Before that some slept on their back and some on their stomach. Fortunately for babies in the USA but unfortunately for some 3 in 2000 babies in the Netherlands at that time the SIDS rate went up in the Netherlands from 1 in 1000 to 1 in 500. Fortunately for future babies that physician and the statisticians in the Netherlands detected the increase in deaths within a year. The physician then studied sleep positions around the world and the rates of SIDS. He noted that in Hong Kong with an excellent health care system and statistical data base the SIDS rate was 1 in 2000 and almost all babies slept on their back. He then got most of the babies in the Netherlands to sleep on their back. The SIDS rate then went down to 1 in 2000. After this was noted and communicated to other physicians in other places tried this same intervention with similar results. After these results were published, some brave physicians in the USA tried the intervention here with favorable results again when the babies slept on their back. By 1991 in the USA it was advised to have babies sleep on their back but with some discretion to the previous tradition recommending sleeping on the side was permissible for physicians who would rather admit to being 90 degrees wrong rather than 180 degrees wrong. By 1999 recommending for babies to sleep on their side was unacceptable as the earlier evidence indicated and it was further confirmed. The USA SIDS rate is now at about 1 in 2500. For more on SIDS see the Nemours site http://kidshealth.org/parent/general/sleep/sids.html and/or the MedlinePlus Site http://www.nlm.nih.gov/medlineplus/ency/article/001566.htm. Through our Public Health Information Technology (PHIT) we must continue to monitor our SIDS and other statistics.

In the mid 1990's some physicians thought that severe forms of breast cancer might be treated with high dose chemotherapy followed by a bone marrow transplant (BMT). This was a time when managed care companies dominated the health insurance market. They and government agencies were refusing to cover the treatment calling it experimental, therefore uncovered by their standard policies. Many patients and their physicians who thought they might benefit from the high dose chemotherapy and BMT after, complained about the lack of coverage. Insurance companies and government agencies asked for more evidence to justify the huge expense of the therapy. Because it was risky and unproven epidemiologist and research oriented disease experts recommended that if the therapy were done, it should be done through randomized clinical trials to best measure if the therapy would really help. If just people who aggressively pursued the therapy were evaluated it might be a peculiar group that might benefit whereas other breast cancer patients with severe disease might fail to benefit due to other unknown or hard to measure factors such as motivation or family support. In April 1999 a nonrandomized study of people who somehow managed to get high dose chemotherapy with BMT for their severe breast cancer. This study failed to show any benefit http://www.stopbreastcancer.org/bin/index2.asp?strid=60&btnid=2&depid=20. By July 2003 two randomized studies also failed to show any great benefit http://www.cancer.gov/clinicaltrials/results/high-dose-chemo0703. Given the high risks, costs, and stress of the therapy without significant survival; physicians and patients now know to avoid such a choice except as the last resort within the context of a clinical trial http://www.cancer.gov/clinicaltrials/digestpage/high-dose-chemo. The insurance companies and government agencies, that discouraged the therapy, were right and the physicians and patients striving to conquer such a terrible disease through the creation of new knowledge were honorable. Patients and physicians just wanting the therapy without improving our knowledge were impulsive, misguided and unrealistic in expecting good results from anything new. Now evaluations and clinical trials are often prohibitively expensive or time consuming to be done to gain more knowledge. With PHIT we may more easily inform physicians and patients of risks and benefits of treatments, we may evaluate treatments and cultural practices, and may more easily and efficiently conduct clinical research for a broad range of conditions and treatments.

There are many more examples of Medical Ignorance beyond the three just discussed. http://www.ignorance.medicine.arizona.edu/. In the 1970's to the 1990's we in the USA were doing more Coronary Bypass Artery Grafting (CABG) than may have been needed. It was a new surgery helping many with clogged arteries with an open chest approach http://www.nlm.nih.gov/medlineplus/heartbypasssurgery.html. It is major surgery with inherent risks. Studies in the late 1970's and early 1980's showed that some people with some types of coronary artery problems did just as well with medications. Now it is used more prudently with more benefits for those getting it; though Dr. David Waters of San Francisco thinks we still do too many surgeries on coronary arteries http://www.businessweek.com/magazine/content/06_22/b3986001.htm. In the 1980's many children got tiny plastic tubes put in their eardrums for ear infections. Later analysis has shown that many children with less severe problems do just as well as those that got the tubes. Now the surgery is used more for those with severe chronic ear problems without response to medical treatment http://www.nlm.nih.gov/medlineplus/earinfections.html; though Dr. Jack Paradise of Pittsburgh believes that we still use too many ear tubes in infants with 300,000 operations per year http://www.businessweek.com/magazine/content/06_22/b3986001.htm. Tonsillectomies were routinely done in the 1930's then with antibiotics in the 1950's done less. Tonsils tend to get larger in children between 6 to 8 years old then smaller after 8 years old http://www.nlm.nih.gov/medlineplus/tonsilstonsillectomy.html. Now we only remove them if they obstruct the airway severely or cause frequent repeated infection. This benefits those with the surgery more and prevents complications from surgery for those who would do fairly well without the tonsillectomy. Still some doctors do it more than others and perhaps to excess. See the work of Dr. John Wennberg on the wide variations in medical practices in different regions of the USA with similar populations http://www.dartmouthatlas.org/. His latest study Dr. Wennberg notes that more care for the chronically ill Medicare population often fails to improve health and does increase costs http://dms.dartmouth.edu/news/2006_h1/ 16may2006_overhaul.shtml. Dr. David Eddy in a *Business Week* interview discusses his work to evaluate medical care using computer simulations. He notes that Britain spends less on health care with better results http://www.businessweek.com/ magazine/content/06_22/b3986001.htm. He lamented that back surgeons thwarted a study to evaluate their operations out of fear of an impediment to do more surgeries; and in a side story at the web site Dr. James Weinstein at Dartmouth notes that in some places physicians do 20 times the numbers of spinal fusions as in other places. Dr. Nortin Hadler of the University of North Carolina believes too many people are getting spinal fusion surgery. These physicians and almost all working in public health economics and health care evaluation agree we need more evidence to help decide what we should do to promote, maintain and/or regain our health. Some of the information is in Evidence Based Medicine (EBM) http:// www.cebm.net/, http://www.york.ac.uk/inst/crd/crddatabases. htm#NHSEED, in the United Kingdom and http://gateway. nlm.nih.gov/gw/Cmd at the National Library of Medicine in the USA. Much of what we do in public health and medicine is unevaluated as Dr. Eddy noted. Some effects that occur only in certain stages of pregnancy may be hard to detect unless specifically examined as with the use of thalidomide that caused severe birth defects http://en.wikipedia.org/wiki/ Thalidomide Using computer models to simulate patients is helpful for designing clinical investigations though computer work must continually be validated with results from patient data and outcomes. What comes out of computers is only as good as what information we give them to work with. People are very complex and we have many genetic and environmental variations that may affect outcomes. Some say about 50% of our health practices are based on custom and tradition. They are perhaps correct but like having babies sleep on their stomachs, using the highest amount of oxygen available for very premature babies, or bone marrow transplants for severe breast cancer we may be incorrect in much of what we do. Using PHIT would do much to continuously gather data on health practices, medical care, outcomes, computer models, and costs to help us make better decisions. The PHIT would help design, administer and evaluate experimental interventions to develop more knowledge.

Physicians and health care providers often fail to do everything that is known that may help the patient. These are medical errors in putting into practice what is proven to work but often lacks significance to the providers and patients. See the AHRQ site for lists of things to do for your and your family's safety http://www.ahrq.gov/qual/errorsix.htm. Many of these practices are simple boring stuff that usually turns out Ok but may lead to adverse outcomes occasionally. For the dedicated health care provider one error is too much and over the year in the USA about 90,000 patients may die from medical errors done in hospitals. The Institute of Medicine discussed this in their book To Err is Human in 2000, and Patient Safety in 2004 with suggested solutions http://lab. nap.edu/nap-cgi/discover.cgi?term=to%20err%20is%20human&restric=NAP. The Institute of Medicine (IOM) [one of the National Academies of Sciences (NAS)] suggests that Electronic Health Record Systems (EHRS's) when properly implemented will help eliminate many medical errors. EHRS's may give physicians, nurses, pharmacists and other health care providers automated check lists and reminders to be sure the basics are done. EHRS's will help legibility and with Clinical

Decision Support (CDS) help deliver high quality information to the health care providers and patients in an efficient manner. "Remaking American Medicine" a TV 4 part series that showed on PBS in October 2006 describes many of the problems and some solutions for current medical care http://www.remakingamericanmedicine.org/index.html. Before the 911 Al Qaeda attack on the World Trade Center we used to think that airplane safety was exemplary. With the pilot and co-pilot going through their safety check lists saying check, check to each other for items that passed inspection. Unfortunately they forgot to put terrorists, extremists or use of airplane as a weapon on their lists, but for the every day things that might go wrong but rarely do this costly time consuming safety work has paid off in eliminating most airplane safety issues that would cost more than the safety procedures. Fred Lee points out that complacency in trained health care providers is the main enemy of competence http://www.pohly.com/books/ifdisney.html. Even if health care workers fail to get paid extra or recognized by the patient for the extra work that they do; they must do the right thing. The ethical strengths of a health care worker have got to be at the top of the list of desirable traits. So far health care payers and patients have failed to fund or do most of these important safety procedures. Electronic Health Record Systems (EHRS) that might automate or make easier these systems are available but currently expensive at $30,000 to $60,000 per physician. Health care payers, governments and patients are unwilling to fund these EHRS that would improve their health and save them money. Some token pilot projects have been done and some insurance companies have given up to $5,000 per physician to subsidize their purchase of EHRS but this is a small start. Physicians that use EHRS in their offices hope to help their patients and are willing to accept less income in the short run. Eventually they may save on record, clerical and administrative costs but the main savings will accrue to the payers and patients who are glad to get these services for free. Insurance company profits and salaries are now showing record highs, but in our capitalist culture this is acceptable as long as the purchasers fail to demand improved safety and efficiency. Now physicians and hospitals get paid more if they make errors, do extra laboratory tests, order more imaging studies, or do unindicated procedures. Patients that get more services generate more billing and thus income with most payment plans. Being more careful may decrease liability costs but often patients or their families will sue if the outcome is poor even though they knew the risks and accepted them. Threats of litigation also incline the physician to order more testing and provide more services even though the benefits are questionable. EHRS with imbedded authoritative clinical knowledge support will help providers make the best decisions with quality improvements and with imbedded payment decision support greater efficiency for patients when the EHRS is based on adequate quality knowledge. If we develop and enable PHIT making it easier for competing insurers and third party administrators to enter the market and to offer better and less expensive plans, we should all benefit. PHIT would pay more for higher quality and more efficient health care saving money that was wasted on disease and disability caused by errors and inappropriate care.

CHAPTER 14
Information Overload:
The Need to Concentrate on High Quality
Information

For those of you taking the short cut from the end of Chapter 3, Know/Hide in Many Ways and the others, I will now try to help us deal with information overload. Even from birth this may be a problem. Brave babies will have their eyes wide open and take in as much as they can while cautious babies will keep their eyes shut and will sleep to avoid information. Sleeping will allow their subconscious to process the information they gleaned from the world. For those of you who are sleeping now after overdosing on this hyperbook and its links, I am happy that your subconscious is processing the information despite the wish by your conscious to forget all this garbage and get up tomorrow to have more sugar, tasty deep fried foods, bask in the warmth of your home territory, and enjoy your new SUV or pick up truck. We all agree that information to warn us of imminent death is important and demands our immediate attention. Fortunately this news is rare in the USA, but then information channels are filled up with things of marginal present significance and/or unlikely long-term effects that may be put there by commercial, political, or academic special interests. I will discuss some rules of information that may help you target in on what is important to you and your community.

The evening TV or radio news, newspaper headlines, or targeted new e-mails often give alerts about violent deaths or injuries of community members. This usually is a simple observational or anecdotal study (1). If we live in the same area and do the same thing we might be at risk also. We might avoid a dangerous road condition or location or some neighborhood at a certain time of day when the violence took place. This might just be a rare occurrence. The same violent event may have not occurred in the same way for 10 or 20 years and it may never happen again. If the injury was caused by ice or by a violent criminal just passing through the area the risk will go down when the causal factor is gone. Even a rare event, if severe such as a fatal motor vehicle injury or a homicide, would warrant caution until the cause of the event was determined.

If we observe the news frequently, our memory may be used to do a simple study and estimate of frequency. The news people, a government agency or a scholar may study the problem and find that the motor vehicle injuries or violent crimes are located mostly in certain spots at certain times we get a better idea of what times and places to avoid in the future. These are the bad parts of town or the bad intersection. This is an association study (2). Statistics may be used to help indicate if the findings are different than a chance or random occurrence. If 20,000 people live in area "A" and 10,000 in area "B" you would expect twice as many injuries in area "A". If 10 times as many injuries occur then statistics will tell you how often that might happen if the events were occurring randomly. Most people start to be concerned or the events are called significant if they have less than a 5% chance of happening randomly (p<.05) http://en.wikipedia.org/wiki/Statistics. The motor vehicle injuries may occur due to high speed limits or limited visibility at an intersection or high traffic for the road design. An association study will fail to tell us that directly. A highway expert might be clued in to studying the intersection based on the association findings and then might predict from other knowledge what might be the problem and suggest a change to the high risk location. If any changes are done the results should be studied to be sure if they were helpful.

If we have a very good memory or if the news people, government agencies, and/or academics keep good records we may plot the occurrence of these violent events by location, time of day, weather conditions and by months or years. We may observe trends over time for different conditions. If the events are common in certain locations and conditions we would be wise to avoid those circumstances. If they are rare and decreasing we should be relatively safe with routine precautions. If we are in an area at times of risk and the events are increasing we should be more cautious and perhaps avoid that in the future. This is a time or trend or historical study (3). These results may also be examined statistically for significance. A criminal expert might say certain robberies in one part of town might be related to drug addiction and note crimes going up with increased money spent on drug purchases. Increased efforts to prevent and treat drug addiction might be suggested along with educating the public on safely protecting their property. Again if an intervention is tried the results should be studied to see if it has any effect.

In the 1920's and 1930's at a Western Electric Company phone equipment Hawthorne manufacturing plant near Chicago, Illinois industrial engineers studied the effect of work conditions on productivity. They increased illumination in the work area, and then noted increased production. This is called an intervention study (4). Being cynical they also tried decreasing illumination in the work area and then also noted increased production. They concluded that the attention that the investigators were giving to the workers inspired the workers more than any effect from the work conditions that they were investigating. This has been called the Hawthorne effect   http://en.wikipedia.org/wiki/Hawthorne effect.   This effect argues for caution in evaluating the results of any simple or single intervention study.

In the 1970's physician studied patients with and without a rare but often fatal disease called Reye's syndrome that causes liver failure after a febrile illness or the flu or chickenpox http://www.nlm.nih.gov/medlineplus/reyesyndrome.html.   At that time acetaminophen (Tylenol) started to be used to help reduce fever in children and infants because it was stable in a liquid formulation. Aspirin or acetylsalicylic acid was used prior to that time. Epidemiologists talked to parents of children with Reye's syndrome, the cases, and children with fevers without Reye's syndrome, the controls. They found that the cases had used aspirin much more than the controls. This was a case control study (5). If this is observed in one study there might be something else that the children or families of the cases are doing different than those of the controls. Aspirin then was less expensive than the acetaminophen so maybe poor kids might get more Reye's than rich kids. The study was repeated often with similar results in both the poor and the rich and both in whites and blacks so we were pretty sure aspirin was the cause. Studies were then done to just have kids use acetaminophen for fevers. The results showed the rate of Reye's syndrome to go down. With this information doctors in the USA began to stop recommending aspirin and other salicylates for children with fevers, chickenpox or influenza in order to avoid Reye's syndrome. It took about 5 years for all doctors to believe the research results and the need to change. The occurrence rate of Reye's syndrome went down for the whole of the USA.

To avoid the problem of the placebo or Hawthorne effect double blind controlled intervention trials (6) are done. From 1985 to 1983 a group of smokers in Finland were given vitamin pills or placeboes that looked exactly alike. The participants and the doctors administering the study were blind to which pills were given to which participants. Often multivariate statistical analysis is used to help determine the significance of these complex studies with many variables http://en.wikipedia.org/wiki/Multivariate statistics. The rate of lung cancer, prostate cancer, strokes and other significant diseases were observed in the study participants. The doctors making the diagnosis of the diseases were also blind to which pills the participant patients were getting. Another investigator getting the information independently from the doctors seeing and treating the patients did the analysis of the results. The effect of getting a placebo or inactive pill could be determined by breaking the code when analyzing the study http://www.cancer.gov/newscenter/pressreleases/ATBCfollowup. The study was done because people who ate diets rich in alpha-tocopherol or vitamin E and beta-carotene had lower cancer rates. Animal studies using vitamin supplements also confirmed the protective and sometimes curative effect of these vitamins on cancer. The results of study showed that those taking beta-carotene had an 18% increase in lung cancer incidence and an 8% increase in overall mortality to the surprise of the investigators. Those taking alpha-tocopherol had 32% less cases of prostate cancer and 41% fewer deaths from it. They also had 50% more deaths from hemorrhagic stroke perhaps from the anti-clotting effect of alpha-tocopherol. Unfortunately for those of you who are picky eaters, just taking alpha-tocopherol and beta-carotene supplements is a poor and sometimes harmful substitute for eating your whole grains, nuts, seeds, and vegetables. More unfortunate for the short-term economically conservative it took about $45 million in 1990's dollars to show that what appeared seemingly obvious failed to work. In the long-term this is a small investment compared with spending resources on vitamin supplements that fail to work year after year. With PHIT the studies may be done with less expense and better analysis. The PHIT may also disseminate the results so that people who are still wasting their money on the wrong nutritional supplements for themselves may stop and adjust sooner.

The double blind controlled intervention trials are quite powerful; though corporations or other groups may provide misinformation by misusing them. Drug companies may sponsor many such investigations using a new drug then them suppress studies with results unfavorable to their new product. When drug companies pay for trials of their new drugs they often have the lead investigators or experts doing the studies sign contracts that allow the drug companies to control the publication or dissemination of the results of the studies http://www.amazon.com/gp/product/0375508465/002-9818530-2024021?v=glance&n=283155. This site contains information on Dr. Marcia Angell's books with reviews and links to other related books. Dr. Angell, former editor of the esteemed New England Journal of Medicine, wrote about this and other misuses of information by drug companies in her books. She and others suggest that there should be a public registry of all drug trials that have been done, are being done and are planned. The registry should also include the statistical results of all the drug trials whether favorable or unfavorable, and then physicians, administrators and patients would have a more true evaluation the drug. Through tax or direct public support we should also encourage direct comparisons of old inexpensive drugs with the new drug, and then we would have enough information to decide if the extra cost and unknown risks of the new drug is worth the price. Now new drugs are often just compared to placeboes yielding little useful comparative information. In the case of Vioxx these comparison studies were inadequate and when the data suggested a problem it was ignored or downplayed by the drug company http://www.fda.gov/cder/drug/infopage/COX2/COX2qa.htm. Vioxx may help some people better than available drugs but it was marketed for everyone without evidence that it was more safe and effective than the standard old drugs for most patients. When a significant side effect such as coronary artery disease occurs there is little justification for using it. In some places health care organizations have used "detail" people to encourage the use of the inexpensive yet effective generic drugs to help save on drug costs. This counters the effect of the drug company "detail" people to encourage the use of their expensive new drugs. With a PHIT integrated with EHRS the latest information on the cost effectiveness of drugs for the patient being dealt with may be delivered to the prescriber in real time. This would include information on what their health care payment plan might cover and on the local availability of the drug. With sophisticated Clinical Decision Support (CDS) drug interactions, allergy problems and dosaging may also be checked. With sophisticated Payment Decision Support (PDS) the patient's co-pay for that drug and the administration of a prior approval application if needed would be done. Sometimes the least expensive and best drug for most people might fail to help this particular patient due to a peculiar allergy, metabolic problem, or drug interaction.

We have good unbiased complete information that will help prevent a fatal disease so now we will change the world, but not so fast. There is the ancient battle between epidemiology and administration, or more broadly put between adapting to threats in the environment and conserving territorial resources. We would like to prevent pain, suffering and the wasting of resources from disease but we need to figure out how to administer the program or treatment, and who will pay for it. Consider meningococcal disease. It attacks about 1,000 youth each year in the USA and kills about 100 http://www.cdc.gov/ncidod/dbmd/diseaseinfo/meningococcal_g.htm. It often attacks college freshmen living in dormitories or recruits in barracks with about 1 case of disease for every 3 thousand freshmen dormitory residents or barrack recruits. The meningococcal germ may spread rapidly in the blood stream causing spontaneous bruising; tiny red spots called petechiae, or bleeding in the skin while incapacitating the heart and kidneys causing death in 10% of the patients if untreated and sometimes if treated with antibiotics within 1 to 2 hours of the first major specific symptoms. If you survive the meningococci invading your blood stream, then it may give you meningitis or an infection of brain. This usually will give you a stiff neck with extreme pain on bending your head even slightly forward. In babies this may make the soft spot or fontanel bulge. In babies and children there is usually a fever also but in teens and young adults fever may be lacking even with the meningitis. The meningococcal germ is surprisingly common with 5% of healthy people carrying it in their throat. The risk of disease is increased when people get a new strain from being in contact with kissing or sharing food or drinks (saliva contact) with large numbers of new people and they get another infection such as mycoplasma (atypical pneumonia or walking pneumonia) http://www.cdc.gov/ncidod/dbmd/ diseaseinfo/mycoplasmapneum t.htm, or cytomegalovirus (CMV) http://www.cdc.gov/cmv/facts.htm or some other infection lowering their immune response and making it easier for the meningococci to invade your throat lining and get into your blood stream. Why not prevent such an awful disease like this? Like anything else it takes time, effort and money to get a vaccine that works, get people to use it and to get resources including money to support the educators, health care workers and vaccine manufacturers and suppliers. In 1978 the military began using a polysaccharide vaccine that worked fairly well for people over 2 years old for 2 meningococcal strains then in 1981 a vaccine for strains A, C, Y, and W was produced. The vaccines were and still are unable to prevent meningococcal strain B that causes about 30% of the meningococcal disease in the USA. With the vaccine costing about $100 per person it would cost $450,000 ($100 times 4,500 people to prevent one death from meningococcal disease from strains A, C, Y and W) if targeting the high-risk group of college freshmen in dormitories or military recruits in barracks. To prevent one death it would cost $4.5 million ($100 times 45,000 high risk people). Most of the disease victims would live and work another 45 years so we might estimate the cost to be about $100,000 per years of productive life gained. For blood pressure control the costs are about $10,000 per year of productive life gained. For the DTaP and MMR vaccines the costs is covered by the savings from decreased medical care so they are cost saving. Prenatal health care saves about 3 times its cost. Insurance companies and most parents were uninterested in paying for the meningococcal vaccine in the 1980's. The vaccine was used if there were an outbreak of a strain of meningococci included in the vaccine with new cases continuing over a week as sometimes occurs. In the late 1980's and early 1990's public support for vaccination of college freshmen living in dormitories increased. Now most college physicians and the National Meningitis Foundation support its use for all new dormitory residents http://www.nmaus.org/about_meningitis/. In the past 2 years there has been a new meningococcal conjugate vaccine that will give good protection from the same 4 strains of meningococci for 8 years instead of just the 3 years with the older polysaccharide vaccine. Since the protection lasts for 8 years and teenagers have some risk even before college the new vaccine is now recommended for teens in the few years before college even down to 12 years of age http://www. immunizationinfo.org/vaccineInfo/vaccine_detail.cfv?id=15 . There as some new vaccines overseas that may work against meningococci strain B but are still far from being used or even tested in the USA http://www.nmaus.org/about_meningitis/. Now some insurance companies will pay for the vaccine and the Federal Vaccine for Children Program does carry the vaccine. If the disease becomes more common or the vaccine cost goes down or if strain B is covered by new vaccines at about the same price then it would be more cost effective with more disease prevented for less cost. With PHIT these factors may be monitored continually in all localities with maximum benefit for the cost of vaccination being obtained. The PHIT may also give patients and their families the latest information on their risks and their costs for the vaccine.

Are we able to save lives and resources on cost saving prenatal care and vaccination with DTaP and MMR? Yes often but the medically indigent, socially disorganized, and stressed families may find it difficult to get prenatal care and vaccination. Medical services to the poor, stressed and disorganized are paid at a low rate through Medicaid or at times without any payment at all, making it hard for providers to get resources to this group that is often more difficult to get to show up for care and to comply with medical directives. Often taxpayers and legislators worry about Medicaid budget problems but in NY State and in many other states 60% of the Medicaid payments go to nursing homes and only 5% go to physicians. We should be sure that any medical care that saves money is given regardless of other expensive programs that it may be associated within the State Budget. Nursing home and elder care may be done more efficiently if it were freed expensive and onerous State regulation with more power and responsibility given to family members to pay and direct the care. President George W. Bush and his administration are encouraging Community Health Centers with cost plus financing to help avoid dealing with getting cost effective health care for all including illegal immigrants. In any other economic sector conservative Republicans would know it would be best to let market forces help distribute the resources. Often Community Health Centers are less productive and fail to serve local communities by simply attracting transient physicians and administrators on salary for 8 to 5 work without helping with emergency, urgent care, or long term needs of the community. These physicians lack territorial interests that help sustain the infrastructure. Fiscal conservatives of any political belief should know that. The Community Health Centers are simply an emergency measure to put off meaningful transformation of healthcare to a system of paying adequately for quality care. For more on giving choice and power to the people in need see Charles Murray's latest book <u>In Our Own Hands</u> <u>http://www.aei.org/publications/filter.all,pubID.24231/ pub_detail.asp</u>. For more on what health care is proven to be cost-effective see http://www.ahrq.gov/ the AHRQ (Agency for Health Research and Quality Web site with links to the US Preventive Services Task Force (USPSTF) and Evidenced-based Practice Centers (EPC's). For a national health plan based on evidence and with the government taking a more active role than Charles Murray would recommend see http://www.radicalmiddle.com/x_health_care.htm. Mark Satin's blog suggest the government direct a rational choice of care for our population. This is logical but will people willingly adopt Dr. Dean Ornish's recommended diet changes or give up expensive futile end of life care for the terminally ill that we now used to having? The government might know best but in the USA we like choice and think, sometimes correctly that we often know better what we need than does some distant bureaucrat. Centralized government control will increase anxiety amongst consumers and providers of health care afraid of under funding of essential services. Charles Murray would have the USA government give every adult $10,000 per year to cover his or her living and health care expenses. If they chose to save money by living healthier and voiding expensive unproven or marginally beneficial health care they would save directly. Public education through PHIT (public health information technology) and other means would be incumbent to create a wise consumer to make this plan work. The mentally ill and mentally challenged without guardians or custodians might need help but others would make their own decisions. PHIT would help in evaluating these interventions in pilot projects in different counties or states to see if we would really improve on our present health care non-system and how best to do it. PHIT might even be used now to see if Health Savings Accounts were helpful and for which people.

Group, local, regional, state, national and world leaders must make tough decisions day to day with the information they receive from within and without. In the examples above we get new information that shows that a change may help our group members but it may be inaccurate or incomplete as with early research showing beta-carotene helping to cure and prevent cancer or that Al Qaeda may have been in Iraq. Our group members may be set in their ways and with limited resources. They may want to avoid the expense and bother of another pill and/or of a large budget item. When the information is solid and is continually confirmed as with seat belts and non-smoking saving lives we know we must act. Newspapers, magazines, radio, TV, Internet, academics, researchers, manufacturers, wholesalers and retailers all have a stake in trying to make new information sound or appear significant to attract us to commercial messages and/or purchase their product. Group members and citizens have inertia to avoid adverse change when things are going well to prevent economic and psychological stress. Fundamentalists and ultra conservatives simply deny anything new is of value and they do well when new information is misleading or seriously faulted. They do poorly however if ignore a real significant danger such as high blood pressure or dangerous driving conditions. Tragic information gaps have happened lately when Louis Freeh the head of the FBI from 1993 to 2001 had an anti-information system bias. When he started as the chief executive of the FBI he had the old computer in his new office removed and never replaced. This was an ominous prelude to the FBI missing the 9/11 2001 plot. President George W. Bush before and after September 11, 2001 wanted to depose Sadam Hussein as the leader of Iraq without bothering to gather enough information to convince our own intelligence staff, our allies and the world of its importance http://www.pbs.org/wgbh/pages/frontline/darkside/. President

G. W. Bush in the past had put more emphasis on social contacts than on information acquisition with his poor academic grades, poor choices of words and improper pronunciations. President G. W. Bush is correct that it is strength to ignore bad information and protect vital territory; but except for extreme fundamentalists and the self-righteous this right of a leader to ignore good information should be severely limited by future voters and other leaders. In his 2004 campaign he and his party claimed this unwavering steadfastness in the face of contradictory truth as strength, labeling his opponent Senator John Kerry as a weak flip flopper for having the capacity to see both sides of an issue and to respond to new information. Senator Kerry and the Democrats also refrained from emphasizing the importance of quality information and analysis. They or some Democratic partisans even may have encouraged some misinformation about President G.W. Bush's service record that in truth was poor but they may have even tried to make it look worse http://en.wikipedia. org/wiki/George W. Bush military service controversy and http://www.nationalreview.com/buckley/wfb200409171421.asp. Senator Kerry's armed service was admirable but his presentation at the Democratic National Convention as being strongly pro-military despite his well know anti-war activities after discharge from the service may have been perceived as moderately deceitful and at least untrue to his character that questioned a problematic war. The more information and Internet savvy frank and truthful candidate Governor Dean was too scary for many of the anxious majority, especially when talking in the vernacular of popular wrestlers and redneck southerners. The anxious may want things better but they are too afraid of major change that may make things worse. It will likely take a more thoroughly educated public with more sophistication in information access and usage through day-to-day access with better systems, to allow politicians promoting unbiased transparent high quality information systems to succeed. President G. W. Bush's controversial use of telephone, Internet and banking records without Congressional or Judicial authorization has likely set back the time table for trust in the security of confidential records for years. The anxious and those in need of extreme privacy and security will be unlikely to divulge their complete health information to any electronic database that might be tapped by federal authorities. The President's admirable effort to make health care better and more efficient through the use of electronic health records is set back by his lack of sensitivity to the privacy and security issues and his lack of judicial consultation http://www.whitehouse. gov/stateoftheunion/2006/healthcare/. The VA's temporary loss of identity information on veterans and the prevalence of cyber crime make many skeptical that our confidential information is presently private and secure http://www.utica.edu/academic/ institutes/cimip/publications/index.cfm. Information systems must prove that they are safe from tampering, unauthorized access, and identity theft; and have limited legally controlled authorized access with clear constraints; and still be useful before the anxious 25% of the population will accept them and the moderately brave 50% of the population would want them.

For those of us with electronic health and business records we are reaping some benefits even now. The separate silos of information with proprietary non-interoperable software make them somewhat difficult to use but it does make them hard to access and resistant to theft. Bill Gates writes about the improved service and efficiencies of electronic information systems that may be achieved now within agencies and businesses http:// www.microsoft.com/billgates/speedofthought/. Now it is possible to have the best information in the world available immediately where and when it is needed or "Just in Time". In June 2006 he writes about trying to unify communications by phone and computer networks to help make communications easier http://www.microsoft.com/mscorp/execmail/. Alvin and Heidi Toffler write about how adaptive corporations and agencies are using information creatively to create new wealth in his latest book Revolutionary Wealth that came out in 2006 http://en.wikipedia.org/wiki/Alvin_Toffler. Newt Gingrich who has worked with the Tofflers has written about some successes in transforming health care with information and corporate changes http://www.cio.com/archive/092203/gingrich.html and http://www.newt.org/backpage.asp?art=2641. Now you may be working on your computer on your office or home network on health or business records and in another window on your computer you may be examining any information on the World Wide Web or Internet. With hyperlinks you may embed the information site into your work so that as the site is updated with new findings your work will also be updated. Data, facts, knowledge and wisdom with known time of creation, quality, bias, and the response of critics may all be accessed for your benefit. If done with a Virtual Private Network (VPN) or with a Secure Socket Layer (SSL) or Transport Layer Security (TLS) the information will also be private and secure http://en.wikipedia.org/wiki/Secure_Socket_Layer. Important information should be stored in encrypted form so that special software and a key or password is needed to access it even if a computer or hard drive, floppy disk or memory stick or card is stolen. The Markle Foundation has guidelines and model contracts to guide evolving networks for health http://www.connectingforhealth.org/ and for public and national security http://www.markle.org/. For important information, such as health or publicly traded securities Sarbanes Oxley Act data http://www.cio.com/archive/070104/sarbox.html, the general information may be provided by a government agency with a details for the public good, a quasi public agency with known standards, and/or a supervised monopoly financed as a utility with user fees.

Without these protections our virtual Internet world is like an undeveloped or third world nation. Viruses, worms, and spyware stream into our unregistered computers used by unknown persons causing havoc at will. Spyware once on a computer may transmit information to other computers without our knowledge. We may use firewalls, antiviral and anti spyware software but often these programs may conflict causing a cyber autoimmune disease that greatly slows and sometimes stops the functioning of the computer. Sometimes we see e-mail or web sites that look like official communications (phishing) but are actually counterfeit and are used to gain our valuable credit card, identity, and password information. This is like drinking contaminated water loaded with germs, living in a community where people lack any accountability for any crimes or traffic accidents, many people have unknown or false identities, and we have to deal with imposters at the bank and market place. In this virtual undeveloped world we try to stay safe in villages of VPN's and SSL's or TLS's with people we know by face and voice. We try to filter out microbes with our firewalls and take antimicrobial medications to combat the parasites that get through but often suffer side effects or drug interactions from the antimicrobial software. Perhaps we should further develop this virtual world with clean filtered streams of information, secure and private identity and information; with strict accountability, and verification of information sources for those that want it. For those that wish to use the Internet as a source of compost for imagination and a relatively safe outlet for primitive behaviors that are dangerous in the public or real world, they might continue to use a primitive form of the Internet that would be monitored to be sure that real vulnerable people are protected. The expression of ideas that might be suppressed by the ruling majority or dominant social groups but that might be adaptive would be a social benefit. Virtual voyeurism, exhibitionism, and sexual behavior between consenting adults that would avoid STI's (sexually transmitted infections) and violent physical confrontations; might be better than prostitution or rape and may more easily be controlled in an anonymous private and secure fashion.

The developed world model for the Internet would filter and purify the information stream, give us locks and keys for our registered virtual homes and thinking machines connected to the information pipeline, and give us effective treatments for any diseases or infestations that might get past these safe guards in the information stream. In developing a more secure, private, and accountable Internet we need to sanitize the pipeline contents to eliminate electronic parasites, give our machines accessing the Internet an identity, give our users (people or cyber agents) an identity, and better test our software to combat viruses, worms and spyware for adverse effects and interactions. With registering machines and users we should also create property rights for virtual space. Theft or destruction of our virtual property should be punishable crimes. In third world development property rights for the poor is an important prerequisite for economic progress http://www.aworldconnected. org/article.php/877.html. Our information should be protected even if residing on other people's systems. It would be like us putting money in a bank. We still own it. The data bank would just be the custodian. We would specify what the bank may do with it and the government would regulate the data banks to be sure the small investors of the public are protected. For very important and private information the government might even be the custodian. The government may access the data in a private and secure manner for public health, public safety or matters of taxation in a transparent and consistent manner. Jim Harper with the Cato Institute suggests that the private sector might do better with controlling identity information in the book Identity Crisis: How Identification is Overused and Misunderstood http://www.catostore.org/index. asp?fa=ProductDetails&pid=1441306. Unfortunately to date the public and private sector have had their problems with identity theft and misinformation. Whatever system is used the guardians of the data much be committed to service and beyond corruption or coercion with the dedication of an elite priesthood. Perhaps a quasi-governmental agency with ample funding and government oversight might work. Intellectual information should continue to be given protection to guarantee rewards to the creators of the information, but we should avoid unregulated monopolies of important ideas that are needed by many in the developing world http://www.infinityfoundation. com/mandala/t_rv/t_rv_agraw_property.htm. Genetic information imbedded in native plants and animals should be owned by the local municipalities where those species reside to avoid corporate piracy by laboratory work http://www.amazon. com/gp/product/0874779537/102-4333282-1841763?v=glanc e&n=283155. The discovery of the genetic sequence may be owned but the gene itself should belong to the ecosystem with the local municipalities as its representative or associate. Similarly basic algorithms, ideas or software useful to all may be in the public domain or when developed by a company government may manage it as a utility or regulated monopoly. Profits would be made within reasonable criteria.

Presently the physician or other health care provider owns the health record. With electronic medical records and detailed comprehensive paper records a great deal of information must be entered. If we hope to make health care more efficient we should take advantage of the 80% of patients or their custodians that would be able to enter their own data. In the future this might be done over a secure Internet connection directly into the patients' individual area in the EMRS (Electronic Medical Record System). Some organizations such as www. RelayHealth.com , www.Medem.org or http://healthvault.com/ offer this service free to patients. With Medem their physicians must pay an annual fee to access the information. Some of the information may be cut and pasted into the EMRS's but most EMRS's lack a direct interface allowing the information to be input into the EMRS's data fields or exported from the EMRS's into the online repositories. Now some and in the future most EMRS will have a private and secure way to give and get information from patients over the Internet. Routine e-mail lacks privacy and security. Web based e-mail with SSL or TLS may be a good way to transmit text. WWW.RelayHealth.com offers this service with a free registration for patients of doctors who have done their free registration also. They offer templates for health messages about specific diseases or symptoms but they charge for that special communication tool with some of the money going to the registered physician for that patient. Presently these on line data repositories are unregulated. Only health care providers are required to keep your records private and secure by law.

If we give the patient ownership of the data as suggested in the above paragraph, the patient may feel more empowered and protected. This may encourage the patient and/or custodian to be more complete and less anxious about data entry. The physician or other health care provider's EMRS's may only have limited access to the entered information depending on the desires of the patient and/or custodian. Teens, who have privacy rights by NY State law but not explicitly under HIPAA, may allow health care providers access to certain information, but may block out their custodian's access in certain circumstances. The teens, adults or custodians may have a PIN (personal identification number) or encoded Identification Card with a picture to give the health care provider of their choice to get access to their records. The EMRS's may store signatures of the custodian, pictures of the patient and/or custodian also for identification and access purposes. The health care provider entering the information would have access to their records for review and management of the patient. Information directly entered by the patient or custodian may be limited to only health care providers specified by them. The patient might limit mental illness or STI (Sexually Transmitted Infection) information to the one doctor in the practice that dealt with that problem and avoid mentioning or disclosing these problems to another practitioner who was just seeing for them for an Upper Respiratory Infection. The patient or custodian would take responsibility for any complications or adverse events occurring that might be due to partial information getting to the provider. The patient or custodian might allow some more information access for life threatening problems such as a heart rhythm problem or severe breathing problems or they may chose to suffer severe consequences if they thought their privacy was paramount. In most EMRS's providers once logged onto the system are able to see all records and all parts of them. HIPAA and State laws simply protect information from disclosure and non-providers of health care. Most EMRS's do track or log anyone that has looked at each section of the patient record but most are now unable to block out certain providers for certain patient. A new generation of EMRS's would be needed to allow for greater patient control of their own data and its access. On-line data storehouses, businesses, and government agencies would be accountable for what they do with your precious information.

Legislation and regulations also play a role in what information is available. In the 1980's many people with AIDS fought and won the right to avoid disclosure of their disease even after they died. In NY State previous to AIDS death certificate information was discoverable for the good of the community but when AIDS was so stigmatizing for families and descendents in the 1980's the courts favored keeping the cause of death confidential with access solely to the Health Department as needed. In the past the Department of Health and courts thought that knowledge of the cause of death by the community would prevent them from worrying about highly infectious diseases such as Tuberculosis and Salmonella. With AIDS just being spread by intimate or blood contacts the general population should have little concern. Now with AIDS and the precursor HIV infection more common and less stigmatizing the NY City Health and Mental Hygiene Department http://www.nyc.gov/html/doh/html/ah/ahb1.shtml and the CDC http://www.cdc.gov/hiv/spotlight2.htm are trying to make testing for HIV infection easier. In the 1980's extensive counseling before and after testing was required in order to advise patients about the implications of testing and the need for confidentiality to prevent adverse social consequences. When we lacked any effective treatment for the disease the testing was of little use except to confirm the grim prognosis. Now with good treatments available too many people are untested early in the disease and often present with severe and sometimes fatal complications. The CDC and NY City would like the test for HIV to be done with a physician or health care providers order without counseling since people already are aware of HIV and AIDS and privacy rights have been recognized. If put in EMRS's this information should be put in the most secure section available on a need to know basis only at the discretion of the patient and/or custodian. Present law allows sexual and blood contacts to be notified of the results but prohibits testing of a patient without consent except with a court order for malignant prisoners. Patients in a coma or who refuse to be tested are a worrisome problem for people who have had blood or intimate contacts with them.

The legislature and the courts may also limit who may be given information and custody privileges. In married couples the spouse of an incapacitated person may get information and make decisions for that person. Health care proxies allow for a formal designation of the person or agent to get information for you and make your health care decisions for you when you are unable to make your own decisions. You may detail your wishes about what types of treatment you would or would not like to have to guide your agent http://www.health.state.ny.us/nysdoh/hospital/healthcareproxy/intro.htm. Simply having a complete and detailed healthy proxy will help prevent pain, suffering and wasted health care if you become unable to decide on your health care and have a terminal illness.

When the logic is uncertain or the science involved in health care or policy lacks consistency and clarity we often go to courts to help evaluate the information. Often courts get cases with bad outcomes regardless of a lack of evidence that any better care may have been given. The plaintiff's attorney simply shows the bad outcome and hopes to persuade the jury that something should be done for the ill or disabled patient. We should have compassion for the ill or disabled, but it should be balanced by our need to maintain territories or infrastructure to help the most people in the community without wasting large amounts of resources on unproven health care or retribution for being unable to prevent or treat a disease without a proven way of prevention or cure. In NY State and many others it only takes one physician with an opinion that the case may have been handled better to get the case to court. The plaintiff may lack any scientific evidence that a better outcome would have been possible. The physician only needs some theoretical or hypothetical guess that one kind of care may have helped that patient. Physicians are a fairly conservative and by inclination try to do every thing practical to help their patients. This good motivation may lead to waste and harm to the patients. In one case of a baby with a stroke a professor suggested that all pale or sleepy infants have a tube put into their trachea (endotracheal intubation) and be given extra oxygen in order to possibly prevent a stroke. About 1 in 4000 newborns have strokes and about 800 in 4000 newborns maybe pale or sleepy in the first few hours of life. About 10% of intubated newborns will get complications with some being fatal. Without controlled clinical trials with repeated success to justify this theory this case should never have gone to court. As we have discussed previously therapies such as extra oxygen for premature babies or extra beta-carotene for smokers may have adverse effects despite some evidence that they might have helped. If we allow anecdotal evidence or simple projections from computer models or animal experiments to direct our care we may be creating more harm than good. The present tort system with mega rewards for plaintiffs and lawyers encourages this. We should ask for quality information such as the double blind controlled trials or intervention studies to be used to guide juries and judges to determine when a court trial is needed. Then the scientific evidence should be carefully evaluated, and the practitioner should be judged on failing to do for a patient what has been proven to work. Philip K. Howard, the founder of Common Good, has suggested that we use Medical Courts to help create and develop judges knowledgeable in medical science http://cgood.org/index.html. His group also would like judges to understand that individual rights must be balanced with community needs in medicine, education and public administration. When we strive to do everything possible to prevent harm and promote well-being for one student, patient or community resident we may actually be over protecting them and creating problems with unwarranted interventions. Even if some good might be possible it might be more harmful for other pupils, patients, teachers, physicians, citizens and communities. The Supreme Court of the USA has given judges the discretion to disallow expert evidence if it fails to meet the criteria of "relevance" and "reliability" http://www.piercelaw. edu/tfield/valdor/valdor.htm . This helps some but in later case reviews the justices have given a great deal of latitude in determining these standards. Professors Kantrowitz and Field have suggested that Science Courts be used for determining controversial scientific policy issues and perhaps tort or liability issues   http://www.piercelaw.edu/risk/vol4/spring/kantro.htm. Some States and the Federal government are now considering legislation to at least try Special Health Courts to see if they would help bring justice to patients and health care practitioners http://cgood.org/f-healthcourtslegislation.html. Whatever ways we use information we will all benefit from improved quality of the information and its rapid accessibility for just in time use with private information only accessed in a secure manner on a need to know basis.

THE WAY
SECTION III

Knowledge Solutions to Balance Territory & Compassion

CHAPTER 15
Continuing Adaptive Behavior: The Way to a Better Life

As we have discussed in this hyperbook, the forces of compassion and territoriality have been fighting it out for the past 2500 years or more. Before that territories and their defenses were a good way to distribute and maintain resources for child rearing and community building. When offensive iron weapons overwhelmed defensive strategies and routine compassion 2500 years ago then more compassion was needed to balance the terrific destruction of strong territorial groups and leaders http://en.wikipedia.org/wiki/Axial_Age. The iron weapons made it easy for powerful territorial rulers and their armies to decimate large populations. This took a lot of the joy out of life and was maladaptive for our species. The compassionate religions of Buddhism, Taoism, Hinduism and Judaism had their roots then, and encouraged the tolerance of diversity to allow adaptation to varying ecosystems with different cultures. This is documented by Karen Armstrong http://www.npr.org/templates/story/story.php?storyId=5307044 . The overwhelming organizational and strategic power of the Roman Empire in public life created more of a need for compassion in private and religious life. The Roman Empire's devastations of non-compliant cultures gave them more resources in the short run but stifled the development of different adaptations to different environments for peoples with different traditions.

The compassion of Christianity helped the people deal with the arbitrary and often capricious rule of distant Emperors with little local knowledge. Mohammed helped the Arabs deal with fractious tribal warfare with respect for life. In the feudal periods stable local territories allowed for local adaptation for survival close to the land or ecosystem. World trade with the exchange of portable territory with goods, jewels, gold and money accelerated in the 1500's with the development of fairly reliable sailing ships in Western Europe. Adam Smith discussed how trade in a free market benefits the buyers and sellers of the virtual territory http://en.wikipedia.org/wiki/Adam Smith. Karl Marx, the communists and socialists responded to the problems of the externalities of free markets- the social turmoil, the disease and the pollution caused by the capitalists' strong hold on their virtual territory http://en.wikipedia.org/wiki/ Karl Marx. In capitalist countries we have tried to temper the free market with social policy, taxation and regulation and in communist countries the ancient need for territories has now been recognized to help give economic stability and efficiency in at least some sectors of the economy. In the energy sector Vijay Vaitheeswaran discusses how market forces regulated for external factors and protection from monopoly may be used to bring greater efficiency to our energy use http://www.amazon. com/gp/product/0374236755/ref=sr 11 1/103-7238491-7920 614?redirect=true&ie=UTF8. Balancing territorial capitalist interests and compassionate humanistic interests is difficult and often perplexing. We now have compassionate capitalists in the USA, and Chinese venture capitalist communists. To further complicate things we have the virtual territorial compassionates who want to help people but only in the way that they see proper. In the intellectual or spiritual realm territorialism may be just as dangerous as in the real world.

These are the self-righteous who believe that they have a monopoly on the way to help the world. When a group believes that they are all compassionate in the only appropriate way and have been correct for 1,000 years they might be called fundamentalists. This is a technique to deal with information overload by discounting all recent information. This is Ok if the new information is of poor quality, but it is maladaptive when things are changing, high quality information is available, and the failure to change may lead to disease and death. We may also have an attachment to physical territory that leads to pernicious combative nationalism and in the future may lead to too much dependence and respect for machines and their evolved state as thinking computers.

Computers will improve over the years with the possibility to reach and exceed human capabilities. Ray Kurzweil and others foresee spiritual machines and transhumans who will be part machine http://en.wikipedia.org/wiki/Ray_Kurzweil. Some of this seems like too much compassion for machines and some of this seems like too much wishful compassion for humans with the machines bringing salvation for incompetent humans and the promise of immortality through a transhuman body http://en.wikipedia.org/wiki/Transhumanism. There are also those who oppose the coming of the thinking computers and transhumans who are known as neo-Luddites http://en.wikipedia.org/wiki/Technological_singularity. They may be seen as protecting the territory of the human species from the invasion and subjugation by machines such as in the movies The Terminator http://en.wikipedia.org/wiki/The_Terminator, A.I. http://en.wikipedia.org/wiki/A.I.:_Artificial_Intelligence, The Matrix http://en.wikipedia.org/wiki/The_Matrix Star Trek: The Motion Picture http://www.imdb.com/title/tt0079945/. In I, Robot humans are able detect problems with the thinking machines before they take complete control. It is based on writings by Isaac Asimov http://en.wikipedia.org/wiki/I_Robot. In I, Robot the artificial intelligence falls into the same territorial trap as humans and becomes self-righteous and violently defensive of its way of helping humans. The development of artificial intelligence will be a challenge for humans. Giving humans strict territorial rights to their data and software may protect us from criminals, invasive business practices, coercive government and invasive competitive artificial intelligence that will be possible within the next 20 years.

Potential disastrous external threats also exist. We have a similar dichotomy of views on extra-terrestrial life with benign or helpful forms as in ET http://en.wikipedia.org/wiki/E.T._the_Extra-Terrestrial, or Contact http://en.wikipedia.org/wiki/Contact_%28film%29; or a predatory form as in Independence Day http://en.wikipedia.org/wiki/Independence_Day_%28film%29 with its software and information battles or War of the Worlds http://en.wikipedia.org/wiki/War_of_the_Worlds_%282005_film%29 with a biologic virus protecting us from susceptible aliens. Should we attract intelligent aliens or hide from them? Attracting extra-terrestrials might bring us helpful new technology and trade to help mankind; but hiding might help protect our territory from advanced predators and complete annihilation of our species.

As we move into the near future we need to adapt by balancing the territorial and compassionate forces as best fitted for our local and global environments. We need information systems to evaluate our problems, create and administer solutions and to evaluate our results on a continuing basis. To avoid the dangers of extreme compassion we must be careful to avoid change based on whims, poor information, self-righteous concepts, or fundamentalist religious or economic principles. We should avoid continuous change in the sense that we change rapidly and immediately at the slightest hint of a problem. Instead we change when we have high quality information or knowledge or wisdom that indicates a significant benefit from a change. May use commonly known management principles to intervene http://emilms.fema.gov/. We respect the local territorial adaptations of an ecosystem and small market that are functioning at present. We respect the intellectual territory of experts who studied the area of change. We would like to avoid changing our immunizations based on introducing a costly vaccine with side effects for a rarely harmful disease, but we would want to adapt quickly to using a vaccine or treatment that would safely save many lives. Our information systems must be timely and have high quality with privacy and security for the protection of individuals and the species.

In the Pre-industrial Age Quality Improvement meant getting more physical territory or land. The Feudal Lords would make a better castle with more surrounding property for defense and sustaining resources. Nations would acquire other weaker less developed nations in imperialism or colonialism. In the Industrial Age or Second Wave Quality Improvement was based on hitting a fixed manufacturing target: getting a high percentage of products to work, getting production of a uniformly sized ball bearing or getting so much production per person. We make our portable and exchangeable territory or goods more marketable. Global trade in products became the new battlefield for nations with trade balances measuring our success. Now with the Third Wave or Post-Industrial Age

Quality Improvement becomes real- time on-line continuous to satisfy the customer with customized use specific knowledge built in. Modern electronic inventory systems note the purchase, track the stock amounts, and place the orders as needed using networks on a just in time basis http://www.microsoft.com/billgates/speedofthought/. Intellectual capital becomes more important. Software, patents, movies, music, books and franchises become important trade items that are now poorly measured and often poorly protected http://en.wikipedia.org/wiki/Alvin Toffler. Our improved productivity may be the result of information systems begun 1 to 7 years ago with intellectual capital built up over time with training, use and familiarity according to studies from MIT http://ebusiness.mit.edu/research/papers/139 Erikb ComputingProductivityv2.pdf. Fred Lee would say in health care as in entertainment, video games and amusement parks, we market an experience rather than a product with the family and the patient's perceptions being our evaluation http://www.pohly.com/books/ifdisney.html. The key to enjoyment in these experiences, family life, and education; is the proper balance of territory and compassion. We expect to give up our portable territory or money to enter the virtual or real territory of the provider of compassionate interactive knowledge that will help our family or primary group to adapt to our real and virtual day-to-day world.

CHAPTER 16
Continuing Quality Improvement for Health

Improving your health starts with you and your family and/ or friends. Nutrition, exercise and social supports happen in your small group of people that you live, work and/or learn with in your primary group. Secondary groups are more formal or institutional http://en.wikipedia.org/wiki/Group_%28sociology%29. Health care work groups or secondary groups work with patients and their primary groups to promote healthier habits and relations. At Dartmouth Medical School these work groups that promote improved health and efficiency are called clinical microsystems http://clinicalmicrosystem.org/. In medical offices, health departments, hospitals, clinics, pharmacies, laboratories and healthcare organizations people want to help their patients to feel better and stay well. When they communicate their observation of problems and their solutions we all gain. When EHRS (Electronic Health Record Systems) with Clinical Decision Support (CDS) and Payment Decision Support (PDS) are introduced into an environment to help the workers to help patients better then better healthcare with greater efficiency is possible. As with any complex systems implementation must be well planned and well supported as in other eBusiness situations as described at MIT http://ebusiness.mit.edu/research/papers-author.html. In the past decade in businesses consultation and education make up about 60 to 70% of the project costs for information systems, with hardware about 5 to 10% and software about 20%. To make systems interoperable the data must be granular; or objective, specific and detailed. If the information system entry says the patient looks well, that is hard to interpret for different people using different systems. The granular entries that might be equivalent would say the patient is content, alert, and clean, has good color, and has good body weight for height. Granular entries may take more time but are more meaningful to more people and easier to transfer to other data systems. Granular data is more useful but is more costly to enter in terms of time of observations done and data entry. As in many businesses with online access patients and their families may do the data entry work for the healthcare provider at their convenience. Practices doing this at present say that 80% of patients provide useful information through data self-entry, though more study is needed. With granular data, symptoms or signs of unknown or unusual diseases (such as possible bioterrorism or emerging infectious disease problems) may be more quickly and better identified and studied.

Even with present regulations and simple data systems we may improve the quality and safety of drugs and biologic agents. Since 1987 the FDA has had authority to document the authenticity of medications. They believe they will have a system in place within the next few years with RFID (radio frequency identification) and/or bar codes http://www.infozine. com/news/stories/op/storiesView/sid/15645/. Hopefully this information may be integrated with EHRS to help healthcare providers better track the use of medications by their patients. The FDA also needs to improve its tracking and supervision of bone and tendon tissue transplants from cadavers http://www. personalinjuryattorney.com/lawyer/transplant_harvested_ body_parts.html. With better tracking the FDA would be able in real time to certify the quality and legality of tissue from cadavers. They would ideally be able to transmit all relevant information to the EHRS of physicians using the tissue in a confidential and secure way.

With an EHRS (Electronic Health Record Systems) with Clinical Decision Support (CDS) the physician may have easily available real time data on the patient's condition; knowledge of the patient's diseases from an EBM (Evidence Based Medicine) data base or other quality information source with recommendations on the current best treatments; information on medications with their adverse effects and interactions; laboratory and imaging results; and reports of consultations from other health care providers. The physician or other provider at the end of the visit may then document the visit and therapies; then transmit that information to other involved providers including consultants, pharmacies and therapists as permitted by the patient or the custodian of the patient. When prescribing medications, studies or therapies the provider may be immediately notified by the EHRS of what the insurance company or payer will cover and what the patient is responsible for. Ideally the provider will be given other options by the CDS within the EHRS for alternate therapies that might be about as equally as effective; and that are covered by the payer, or that are more economical to the patient. With an EHRS with PDS (Payment Decision Support) the patient or their custodian may find out at the time of signing in for their health care what their insurance status is and what services it will cover for that office or clinic visit. PDS will also help the provider determine if they will get paid by a third party payer (insurance or government or no-fault or workman's compensation, etc.) and how much prior to the visit. The EHRS with PDS may help patients, employers, third party payers, and public health evaluators determine how much we spend for what services and what we get in terms of outcomes or success in promoting health, treating disease, and recovering health in real time. The PDS may also help payers administer their payments more efficiently based on providers meeting safety and quality standards. This is commonly called "pay for performance". Now most "pay for performance" or "P4P" are hard to administer with paper records and often just give payers an excuse for taking away payments from physicians who provide more though perhaps better services to their patients. Before we get good enough to know what best is in healthcare at least we may pay providers for provider data in a useable form with "pay for participation".

The PDS (payment decision support) would also help patients and purchasers through government evaluations and/or standards to find the most efficient payers or insurance companies. The payers may be evaluated for the products producing the best health outcomes for the least amount of cost. Now payers often get paid more to spending more money since most large corporations are self-insured. The payers then act as a Third Party Administrator (TPA). The TPA's often get paid a percentage of the payments they make to providers, so the more services they pay for the more money they get. Many insurance companies act as TPA's and use the same antiquated data systems that they use for their insurance payments to providers. The large employers who use TPA's are often kept uninformed of the nature, amount for specific health care, and specific problems treated. The TPA's thus often prevent competition from other TPA's since they own the data and fail to share it with the purchaser. Other TPA's then are unable to bid competitively since the have too many unknowns in their estimates. With EHRS containing PDS with PHIT, the purchasers of health care, payment services, and insurance would be better able to evaluate what they were getting. These interoperable administrative and data systems with public supervision and guaranteed private and secure access may also be used for new payers to more easily enter the market. Now competition into markets is often cost prohibitive due to the initial price of data and administrative systems. Payers and insurers now have a near monopoly or oligopoly with excessive economic power over the providers. The combined EHRS with CDS and PDS within PHIT networks would give the market more elasticity for the provision of payment services. Services to prevent or control: diabetes, high blood pressure, smoking, and safety problems may be rewarded if they work to help improve health in an efficient manner. Local programs may offer services tailor made to deal with local problems and to use unique local health care providers. Savings in such a system comes from avoiding duplicate care (office visits, medications, laboratory tests, imaging studies, and therapies) from different providers and progressing more quickly to better care or recognizing more easily that everything practical has been done. Health care proxies or living wills for terminal or hospice or comfort care patients would be easily accessible allowing for a dignified and compassionate end of life without wasting undesired resources just to avoid litigation. The patient would save their time and energy and the payers would get fewer bills. Medication and test cost would go down for most patients with generic drugs and a limited amount of tests done based on EBM (Evidence Based Medicine) knowledge embedded in the system. Unless compensated for the EHRS with CDS and PDS, the provider would get less money. The Office of the National Coordinator for HIT (ONCHIT) estimates that such a system would cut our health care costs by 20% with the most savings going to the payers and most costs to the providers http://www.hhs.gov/healthit/valueHIT.html. This easily explains why progress for health care providers in implementing HIT is so slow. Only a self-sacrificing quality obsessed physician or administrator with available financial resources would be interested.

One way to help the patient and their family get savings from more efficient health care is by using Health Savings Accounts (HSAs). The HSAs must be used with a qualified high-deductible health plan (HDHP). The patient and/or family put the deductible amount into the HSAs with pre-tax income. The family or patient may use the HSAs to pay any qualified health expenses http://www.nahu.org/legislative/MSAs/HSAs-HSSAs/index.cfm. Interest on the HSAs accrue tax-free and accumulates each year if unspent. The HSAs are transferable from job to job and maybe used by the self-employed. Here is an example of one plan offered by one insurance company http://www.health—savings—accounts.com/golden.htm. These often help middle and upper class families and patients but often unaffordable to low-income groups. Information on costs of services must now be gathered by the patient or their custodian, but this activity will help them appreciate the services more appropriately than if someone else were paying the bill. Alvin Toffler might call this prosumption http://en.wikipedia.org/wiki/Alvin Toffler—the consumer now doing the work that the payer or insurer would be doing. Some people call this consumer-oriented health care. If we wish to continue with the capitalist model of health care delivery we should make sure the market values and options are perceivable by all consumers to help them make the best choices for themselves. This makes the market transparent to the buyer. The EMRS with PDS and CDS for the patient or family might be used to give the consumer an efficient, private and secure way to comparison shop and perhaps purchase health services such as medical care, drugs, therapies and diagnostics on the web through a PHIT. Patients, consumers and payers may then do "P4P" (pay for performance or efficiency) for healthcare payment administrators and insurance companies.

The main question now is how we should motivate patients, their families and their healthcare providers to implement and to pay up front to gain future savings from the EHRS (Electronic Health Record Systems), CDS (Clinical Decision Support), PDS (Payment Decision Support), and PHIT (Public Health Information Technology) to link patients, providers and RHIO's (Regional Health Information Organizations) or SNO's (Sub Network Organizations). To improve the quality and efficiency of health care we must first plan our system and its implementation, then we may encourage health care payers with extra money to invest in PHIT since they will save the most money but the State should set the standards for the functions and specify that all qualified state residents, providers, payers, patients, and administrators are able to use the private and secure health information system. For-profit companies might get a short-term tax break to help with startup costs and not-for-profit companies might one time grant to help out until the savings start in 1-3years. The increased elasticity in the entry of new payers and the increased transparency in the market should help give savings back to the State and its residents. Some start up temporary funding might also be justified since some payers investing in provider HIT might lose market share and some might gain. Using present market share might cause unfair subsidies to low current market share companies that expand in the future. In a second way, the State might pay providers directly the start up costs for their HIT and just have the payers pay for their hardware that would run the specified interoperable standard software. Participation in State plans; such as Medicaid and/of Medicare; might be required. Providers or payer may be able to add on to their software as long as it met the minimum specified standards for quality, accounting and interoperability. The payers, according to how many of their patients the provider saw, might pay the yearly costs. In a third way, the State might provide basic open source software that would work on low cost hardware and networks; and might be added to by private vendors. The providers and payers would cover the hardware and Internet costs. Combinations of all 3 ways might also work with careful planning. The State's residents should save on health care costs, gain in quality of health and perhaps spend more on other goods and services. Businesses would be able to generate more revenues and taxes. Decreased costs of living and doing business in the State would attract more residents and visitors. The State would eventually be able to save operating expenses by using the health information system to replace and expand its antiquated and isolated health data systems such as SPARCS of NY State (a data base of hospital admissions), birth records, death records, infectious disease reporting, laboratory reporting, birth defects reporting, the Newborn Screening Tests, community health care, home nursing services, nursing home reviews, hospital reviews, lead reports, restaurant reports, water reports, mosquito reports, zoonoses reports, biohazard reports, and environmental reports. Contacts with health care providers and residents would be private, secure and customized to the immediate needs our residents. Providers and community members would easily be able to report problems and get responses without aggravating territory holders unnecessarily.

CHAPTER 17
Creating Balance between Compassion and Territory

Now all we need to do is to use quality information to help balance the ancient vertebrate trait of territoriality, manifested in anxiety, depression and conservatism; and the ancient trait of compassion manifested in empathy, humanism, intellectualism, and socialism to help make our society more adaptive. Niccolo Machiavelli tells us about the hazards of advocating for change in The Prince, "And let it be noted that there is no more delicate matter to take in hand, nor more dangerous to conduct, nor more doubtful in its success, than to set up as a leader in the introduction of changes. For he who innovates will have for his enemies all those who are well off under the existing order of things, and only lukewarm supporters in those who might be better off under the new. This lukewarm temper arises partly from the fear of adversaries who have the laws on their side, and partly from the incredulity of mankind, who will never admit the merit of anything new, until they have seen it proved by the event." http://en.wikipedia.org/wiki/The_Prince#External_links. Health insurance companies, Workman's Compensation insurers, physicians doing well with the present insurance system, State and private administrators and bureaucrats, malpractice lawyers, vendors supplying the health care information technology sector in its present form, and state legislators benefitted by the present infrastructure all may be threatened by change in Public Health Information Technology that works to improve quality and efficiency. Alvin Toffler sees many industries racing ahead to adapt to our new information technologies and its accompanying culture of the post-industrial state or third wave, but many bureacracies, in the private and public sectors, will resist to the detriment of our ability to survive in a rapidly changing and competitive world http://en.wikipedia.org/wiki/Alvin Toffler. Joseph Campbell would describe this inertia as the dark force that must be overcome by the hero to redeem the world or at least let it adapt http://www.jitterbug.com/origins/myth. html. George Lucas would cast it as the Dark Side of the Force with anxiety and fear. Colin Campbell notes the resistance in the medical establishment and food industry to trying out the whole food plant derived diet www.thechinastudy.com. In NY State Mark Bitz is attempting to overcome a whole infrastructure of political inertia well described at his web site and in his book Creating a Prosperous New York State http://www.freenys.org/index.php. We might call it "the Empire State takes a pre-emptive strike at change" and how to overcome it with a heroic effort. He does endorse using information to evaluate the functions of the State including its schools and economic health to help decide what to do. He would like to eliminate gerrymandering or strange election districts to help guarantee success for incumbents. This is a major problem in NY and many other States of the USA. For an impartial redistricting plan we might use Cluster Analysis or a geographic multidimensional statistical analysis with the voters deciding what variables are most important. Should we emphasize physical geography such as valleys, rivers and mountains; traditional minor civil divisions such as counties, towns, villages, and cities, school districts, ethnic groups, religious groups, or areas of commerce; or any combination http://www.statsoft.com/textbook/stcluan.html, http://en.wikipedia.org/wiki/Cluster_analysis? In April 2007 Governor Elliot Spitzer formed The Commission on Local Government Efficiency and competitiveness chaired by former Lieutenant Governor Stanley Lundine that may help the transformation of NY http://www.ny.gov/governor/press/0423071.html. In the nation we may use a national defense and/or community service program to help reach common goals http://www.beliefnet.com/story/135/story_13586_1.html as suggested by Frank Schaeffer. In the international arena might follow the example of the group called "For the Common Good" http://www.commongood.info/. They try to be spiritually and culturally sensitive to the developing the world when promoting international communications and trade. In health and energy development we may use regulated market forces to help get the best results for our resources as suggested by Vijay Vaitheeswaran in <u>Power to the People</u> with decentralized power helping PHIT stability http://www.amazon.com/gp/product/0374236755/ref=sr_11_1/103-1733450-9433442?ie=UTF8. In all matters we should seek high quality information or truth to help when territory and compassion conflict as Mahatma Gandhi did to resolve disputes http://en.wikipedia.org/wiki/Mahatma_Gandhi. When choosing political leaders, group leaders, organization members and co-workers we should give preference to those who are able to give us the best information regardless of whether or not it favors their preferred beliefs or theories. This should help our society and groups be more adaptive to reality and give us a better chance to succeed in times of limited resources.

The arts help us deal with compassion and territory. Two musical plays and the responses from 1957 NY City tell us about our humanity and culture. In <u>The Music Man</u> the salesman Harold Hill provokes territorial defense of the community from pool playing by boys to sell his band instruments and uniforms for the boys <u>http://en.wikipedia.org/wiki/The_Music_Man</u> . The compassion of the adults for the boys in their fancy uniforms then protects him from buyer's regret or anger for his poor capabilities in teaching music. He tries to be friendly with the local politicians, youth leaders, and the music teacher to allow the home and musical territory to be entered. Other salesmen feel their work territory and sales being threatened by his lack of technical and geographic knowledge and would like him to leave their marketing area. He usually gets out of town before the adults realize what has happened but in the town of River City he gets emotionally involved with the librarian Marian and her younger brother. Fortunately the band gets dressed up and figures out to how play some before his public inquisition takes place. In the same year <u>West Side Story</u> came out with a NY City musical version of Romeo and Juliet in which 2 lovers try to overcome the hostility of their fighting territorial groups: the Sharks and the Jets <u>http://en.wikipedia.org/wiki/West_Side_Story</u>. They fail to prevent some death but by their compassion they help both sides to recognize the humanity of the other group. The TONY Award for best musical for the 1957 to 1958 season went to <u>The Music Man</u> <u>http://www.tonyawards.com/en_US/archive/pastwinners/index.html</u> . This may have been recognition of the importance of advertising and corporate formation for the economy of NY City and a desire to try to escape the depression of entrenched territorial conflict with zero sum games <u>http://en.wikipedia.org/wiki/Zero-sum_game</u>. Similarly in IT and social change forming trusted friendships, getting adequate funding, and picking good group leaders is better than fighting tooth and nail for limited resources within an organization.

We must be grateful for Bill and Melinda Gates' work in global public health and disease prevention with their Foundation http://www.gatesfoundation.org/default.htm . Their new knowledge in viruses, parasites and bacteria and the human immune system will help world health. They are helping to deal with common diseases and improve basic pregnancy and delivery care around the world. They are also helping improve education in the USA with motivation and resources. This work may also help Bill Gates direct Microsoft to better security from virtual worms and viruses, to help develop a better immune system for computers and networks, and to better educate us on the using technology to help our species adapt.

We must avoid the territorial blunder that all information systems are good. We should recognize the comedy of PHIT (Public Health Information Technology). Comedy occurs when a logical behavior is seen as maladaptive. Puns sound right but mean wrong. Slapstick shows common human behaviors in the wrong context bringing ridiculous consequences. Old manners and habits become strange and malfunctional in a new world. Information systems though well intentioned, if poorly designed or poorly implemented or poorly funded will cause more harm than good. Here are some of PHIT's bloopers. In Syracuse, NY in the late 1990's Crouse Hospital went into bankruptcy briefly when their information system failed at billing correctly and promptly http://www.hfma.org/publications/know_newsletter/051706.htm. NY State Empire Health Insurance nearly failed when their Board of Directors tried to bring on cutting edge information technology that was apparently unready for prime time data processing. In NY State the Department of Social Services in the 1990's lost $200 million on a failed data mega system implementation. At

Cedars-Sinai Hospital in Los Angeles the implementation of their medical record system failed when it took too much time and effort from their physicians http://www.washingtonpost. com/wp-dyn/articles/A52384-2005Mar20.html.   Physician time is valuable for gaining payments and for helping care for very sick patients. Time pressure perceived or real is very threatening to physicians in private practice. It is their home territory that they fight tooth and nail to protect. Dr. D. Brailer notes that about 1/3 of health information technology (HIT) implementations fail. Information technology (IT) with poor motivation will fail society even if it technically succeeds such as Hitler's use of data cards and IBM machines to track minorities and the disabled in order to move them to concentration camps or institutions http://www.ibmandtheholocaust.com/ home.php. This is very dark humor in IT but it warns us to avoid IT without the safeguards of public control of security and privacy with guaranteed minority rights. In Pittsburgh the University has had possible problems in implementing their computer order entry systems http://www.post-gazette. com/pg/06169/698983-28.stm. Physicians are anxious about possible disruptions in patient care and physician schedules. At the University of Pennsylvania the Computerized Physician Order Entry System created new types of errors http://www. cio.com/archive/060105/tl healthcare.html.   Generally,   the larger the project is the more likely the failure is. PHIT and IT projects are best done gradually in small pieces over time with much training and guidance. PHIT is a tool to help people work better to help others. Worshipping PHIT, HIT or IT might become another dangerous fundamentalist religion with more harm than good or another addiction in need of a re-orientation to the higher goal of species adaptation with the 12 steps to escape technology and junk information addiction http://en.wikipedia.org/wiki/12 steps.

For humans to adapt to our world, we must conserve our human resources by using them wisely to help the most people. For this we need high quality information. We should allow our species to develop its potential through a civil diverse equitable society that produces high quality information and disseminates it while preserving the environment that we depend on. We may have many theories of how best to distribute wealth and other resources such as capitalism, socialism, compassionate capitalism, conservative socialism or pragmatism. We should all agree that whatever we try we must continually evaluate it and adjust our behavior depending on what kind of results we get. Work that helps others and creates efficient technologies should be rewarded. We must resist too frequent or confusing change, yet promote needed adaptation and adjustments when truly needed. I think we would all agree that we need open public information systems to do these evaluations, communicate results, get responses from our residents and citizens; and then plan to intervene to improve our community, State, nation and world. Our institutions of religion, education and politics should be continually seeking quality information and adjusting their adaptive programs to the benefit of our species. Religion at its best seeks to help the poor and depressed of the world with compassion and understanding. Identifying their problems accurately and helping those with the greatest needs when possible should be a top goal to help social stability and security while preserving efficient infrastructure that already helps many people. As with other projects we need quality information on religious and ethical problems, their possible solutions, and the results of applications of these solutions to avoid defensive responses from nationalism and self-righteousness. Information about and sensitivity to traditional territorial educational and economic solutions is important even if these systems have failed since rapid changes without respect for people and their traditions will create anxiety and violent defensive response. At its best education informs what is known and learns more from its students and research on their world. Quality and efficiency in information is the basis for education and its transformation for our population and the professions. The open political process informs politicians and the public about their needs, ideas and how they would like to adapt. Good politicians and citizens seek quality information and inform the voters on what may be done and how they would like to do it. A good political debate should encourage quality information systems, publicize the best information available and allow the voters to chose what action they believe is most likely to help them. Once a program or project is done we start all over again to see if the intervention has had any effect and see how it is helpful and/or harmful, educate the public, and reiterate the process in a continuing manner. With information technology that is secure and private for individual data, yet transparent and accessible for community and public data we have a chance to adapt our species to our world and perhaps beyond.

In my career in public health the territorial often beats the compassion since most politics is based on territory. In the 1970's the Democratic Machine in Albany County cringed when I released infant mortality data to the public Health Systems Agency. Then as now poor people living in poor areas have much higher infant death rates than those well to do people living in the elite suburbs. I was expelled from the local health department. The Commissioner of Health of the State of NY Dr David Axelrod did note that the information was public. More on this in my upcoming book <u>Up From Intelligence</u>.

The Democratic Machine also gave the local Albany Medical College Pediatrics Department resistance in trying to eliminate the chronic lead poisoning problem in the old Albany town houses covered with Dutch Boy lead paint made by National Lead. Significant territory should be protected but if it is ill and maladaptive it will become worthless.

In the immediate future our human, culture, science, paper, electronic and computer information systems should address how best to prevent if possible: catastrophic climate changes, the toxic effects of the rich Western diet, the negative health effects of smoking cigarettes and the use of other addictive drugs, the dependence on oil and fossil fuels, the lack of exercise in Western type societies, the use of violence to deal with social problems; and the effects of past, present and future infectious disease of humans and computers. I would suggest that try approaches best suited to local geography and culture. For most people, we should try to eat a whole food plant based diet, exercise regularly in a way to create storable energy or avoid the use of fossil fuels, work to understand health and social problems to deal with them before people feel severely threatened, and promote all people working together to advance the stability and diversity of our species on our home planet and perhaps beyond. All interventions or changes would be administrated by our information systems and monitored for their effects on territories and people in their biosphere. Future changes will be planned using the continuing flow of information with objective transparent yet private and secure evaluations.

THE DISCUSSION CONTINUES

For corrections, suggestions and addendums please e-mail me, Phillip Gioia. If you permit I will attach your contributions to future electronic copies of this hypertext.

Secure e-mail at www.RelayHealth.com—a free registration is required. Insecure e-mail drgioia@verizon.net

Web site with general health information and contacts—http://pages.prodigy.net/pcgioia

Made in the USA
Charleston, SC
31 October 2010